on Jan 28 my
66th B-Day - Lucy
Nancy while we
were having
lunch.

AYURVEDIC SECRETS TO LONGEVITY & TOTAL HEALTH

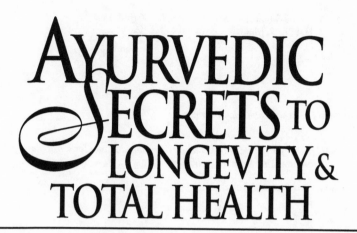

PETER ANSELMO WITH JAMES S. BROOKS, M.D.

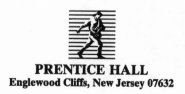

PRENTICE HALL
Englewood Cliffs, New Jersey 07632

Library of Congress Cataloging in Publication Data

Anselmo, Peter.
  Ayurvedic secrets to longevity and total health / Peter Anselmo
with James S. Brooks.
    p. cm.
  ISBN 0-13-156432-3 (case).—ISBN 0-13-156465-X (pbk.)
  1. Self-care, Health. 2. Medicine, Ayurvedic. I. Title.
RA776.95.A55 1996
615.5'3—dc20   96-2833
                                                        CIP

Printed in the United States of America

10 9 8 7 6 5 4 3 2 1

ISBN 0-13-156432-3 (c)   ISBN 0-13-156465-X (p)

This book is reference work based on research by the author. The opinions expressed herein are not necessarily those of or endorsed by the publisher. The directions stated in this book are in no way to be considered as a substitute for consultation with a duly licensed doctor.

PRENTICE HALL
Career & Personal Development
Englewood Cliffs, NJ 07632
A Simon & Schuster Company

On the World Wide Web at http://www.phdirect.com

Prentice Hall International (UK) Limited, *London*
Prentice Hall of Australia Pty. Limited, *Sydney*
Prentice Hall Canada, Inc., *Toronto*
Prentice Hall Hispanoamericana, S.A., *Mexico*
Prentice Hall of India Private Limited, *New Delhi*
Prentice Hall of Japan, Inc., *Tokyo*
Simon & Schuster Asia Pte. Ltd., *Singapore*
Editora Prentice Hall do Brasil, Ltda., *Rio de Janeiro*

CONTENTS

Chapter 15—"Don't Worry, Be Happy" — Ayurvedic Secrets for Overcoming Anxiety   214

Chapter 16—How to Keep Your Cool— Ayurvedic Strategies for Mastering Anger   225

Chapter 17—Ayurvedic Secrets for Fulfilling Relationships   236

Chapter 18—Sex and Your Constitutional Type: Ayurvedic Secrets for Intimacy and Fulfillment   254

INTRODUCTION

The principles and practical techniques in this book are derived from Ayurveda, the ancient system of natural medicine from India that is undergoing such a wonderful revival throughout the world today. The healing techniques and preventive methods of Ayurveda include:

- personalized dietary recommendations for health, balance, and vitality
- daily routines designed to take maximum advantage of nature's rhythms
- stress management and meditation to settle the mind and relax the body
- simple exercises to increase energy, promote strength and suppleness, and increase mental clarity
- an oil massage we can give ourself in less than ten minutes to nourish and soothe the nervous system and increase mental and emotional centeredness
- herbal food supplements to help us access our body's innate healing intelligence, strengthen the immune system and bring balance to mind and body, and much, much more.

Ayurvedic healing methods are not designed primarily as "magic bullets" just to wipe out symptoms. Rather, they promote wellness by steadily building mental, emotional, and physical strength. They are entirely natural and gentle and involve no synthetic drugs with their potentially harmful side effects.

These methods are enjoyable in themselves and produce relaxation, energy, and increased joy of life. Because of their safety and effectiveness, they are being prescribed and recommended for both prevention and healing by increasing numbers of physicians, therapists, and other health professionals all around the world.

This book brings the core knowledge and practices of Ayurveda directly to you. With the information in this book, you will be able to create real changes in your life in a very short time.

At the beginning of the book, you will learn how to determine your constitutional type, your own nature according to Ayurveda. Armed with that understanding, you will be able to select the diet, exercise program, herbal supplements, and other keys to health that are suitable for you *and use them on your own*. In short, this book will give you the tools to create a state of physical, mental, emotional, and spiritual health and balance. It is meant to empower you, to give you more control over your own life and health. Use it to create and maintain a high level of wellness and well-being.

What This Book Will Do for You

If you are a fundamentally healthy person, but wish to rid yourself of the occasional colds, low moods, worries, and minor ills of ordinary life such as sleepless nights, digestive upsets, and other stress-related problems, the knowledge in this book will help you quickly move up to radiant good health.

If you are struggling to get free of a chronic illness or condition, or are battling destructive or self-destructive behavior such as addictions, eating disorders, or outbursts of anger, Ayurveda offers you simple, effective tools to gain more control over your life.

Even if you are in the grip of a more serious illness, the knowledge and techniques of Ayurveda may bring you relief from your symptoms and set you on the path to full and lasting recovery. Ayurveda combines extremely well with most standard Western medical procedures. With the cooperation of your physician, you may, over time, be able to reduce your need for medications.

If you are in the recovery stage, healing the wounds of a serious illness, childhood abuse, alcohol abuse, divorce, or any painful loss, you will find the Ayurvedic techniques, such as meditation and massage, remarkably soothing, healing, and strengthening.

And if you are a health professional, you will learn principles and practices that you can put to use every day, both to maintain your own health and balance in the midst of the stress of your profession and to offer to your patients and clients. You will be deeply gratified to participate in their real and lasting recoveries.

Women and men of all ages and backgrounds who apply Ayurvedic principles and techniques in their lives enjoy not only vastly improved physical health, but an unfolding of self-esteem, inner joy, peace, and stability. Outwardly, they become more dynamic and effective in action. Inwardly, patience and love seem to develop without effort, and relationships improve. These benefits have helped tens of thousands of people over the last couple of decades as Ayurveda has become increasingly well-known in the West.

An Overview

Part I will quickly introduce you to some of the fundamental principles of Ayurveda that you will need in order to use the rest of the book. You will also take a brief self-evaluation that, along with the principles, will help you discover and understand your constitutional type.

Part II offers six key strategies for building perfect health. You will learn how to strengthen your immune system and how to use diet, exercise, herbal supplements, stress-management techniques, and daily and seasonal routines to organize your life for maximum health.

Part III presents strategies for preventing and healing common health problems and concerns such as colds, digestive difficulties, insomnia, PMS, fatigue, weight problems, and so forth.

Part IV is dedicated to developing greater mental and emotional wellness and enhancing relationships. Here you will learn some powerful Ayurvedic insights for improving intimate love relationships. You will also learn how to deal better with depression, anxiety, and anger. Young couples will find helpful suggestions in the chapter on pregnancy and prenatal and infant care.

We will conclude with a vision of a healthy world, brought about by applying Ayurvedic principles of prevention and healing in our lives.

A final word: You may encounter some new ideas in this book and some new terminology. Don't feel you have to incorporate all these principles and suggestions into your life overnight. But please—don't just read the book and go away! Even one or two of these techniques will make a big difference in your life.

Put them to work! You will notice major improvements in your health and well-being, and the purpose of preparing this book will have been fulfilled.

PART   1

AYURVEDA
AN ANCIENT SCIENCE
REBORN

AYURVEDA
AN ANCIENT SCIENCE REBORN

Ayurveda is considered by most medical historians to be the world's oldest system of natural medicine, originating at least 3,000 years ago. Many of the other ancient systems of natural medicine, such as Egyptian, Chinese, Persian, and Greek, are believed to have their roots in Ayurveda.

The word *Veda* means knowledge or science. The vast Vedic literature of India, often referred to as *Vedic Science,* contains detailed knowledge about the laws of nature and their application to human life.

Ayus means life or life span. *Ayurveda* is thus the "Science of Life" or "Knowledge of the Life Span." It deals with the fundamental principles in nature that underlie the creation, preservation, and restoration of health and the promotion of longevity.

Ayurvedic medicine is a complete science of healthy, balanced living. It is a genuinely holistic knowledge, encompassing the whole range of life, inner and outer.

A Holistic System of Health and Longevity

Ayurveda is holistic in many ways. First, it views the individual as an integrated whole, not just as a collection of parts requiring specialized attention (eyes, lungs, heart, etc.). It also sees the person as

7

intimately connected to nature and the universe. Your environment, relationships, job, and constitutional type, your diet and activities, even the weather and the season of the year—all these are important, and all are taken into account for prevention, diagnosis, and treatment. Mind, body, and Self—mental, physical, emotional, and spiritual—are all included in Ayurveda.

Ayurveda views each and every person as unique, with a unique mind-body constitution and a unique set of life circumstances, all of which must be considered in determining either natural healing approaches or recommendations for daily living.

The theoretical side of Ayurveda provides insights into how to live one's life in harmony with nature and natural laws and rhythms. Its practical side—especially its guidelines for an intelligently regulated diet and daily routine, its techniques for stress management, and its exercises for increased fitness and alertness—help us take control of our lives and develop radiant health.

The central goal of Ayurveda is nothing less than a state of perfect health, for the individual and for society and the environment as well, in which every man and woman is inwardly in balance and outwardly in harmony with the environment and the laws of nature.

A System of Natural Medicine

To say that Ayurveda is a system of natural medicine means something a lot more profound than that it uses natural herbs and natural procedures, such as breathing and stretching exercises, to promote health.

According to Ayurveda, nature is permeated by intelligence. Intelligent laws govern the growth of all living things; kittens grow into cats, acorns into oak trees. Indeed, laws of nature regulate everything, from the tiny world of whirling atoms to the huge, enormous world of galaxies.

The human body is part of nature—a magnificently designed part—and when it runs perfectly, as it was designed to run, it can be perfectly healthy. It is *trying* to be perfectly healthy all the time, using its innate self-healing, self-regulating ability as it strives for a perfect homeostatic balance. But we repeatedly interfere.

It is much more difficult to violate a law of nature than to live in accordance with it. Swimming downstream, with the current, is easier than swimming upstream, fighting the current. The current of life carries animals to sleep at dusk and awakens them at dawn, it creates mating seasons and mass migrations, it makes all things grow and evolve according to their own nature.

What could be simpler than just being what you are, being in touch with your nature? And yet we get out of touch.

In our modern way of life we have done so many unnatural things, adopted so many unnatural lifestyle patterns, that we have thrown off the natural intelligence of the body. We have gotten ourselves out of balance, through wrong diet, underexercise or overexercise, negative thinking, accumulating stress and fatigue, watching violent movies, and so on. And unfortunately, once we are out of balance, it is not hard to get worse.

Once you're out of touch with that flow of nature, the "mistake" easily proliferates. If you're feeling dull from drinking too much alcohol, you have some caffeine to wake you up. One violation of natural law—of what is good for you—leads to another.

Nature has set us up with all the equipment we need to be perfectly healthy. It sounds almost silly to say so, but health is our natural state, and ill health is unnatural. Every day our systems are exposed to literally millions of bacteria, viruses, allergens, even carcinogens, and yet our immune system has the intelligence and skill to deal with all those invaders and keep us healthy. However, when stress, inadequate nutrition, or just fatigue weaken the immune system, those same invaders may produce disease.

Every second the body is adjusting to countless thousands of changing parameters, keeping us in homeostatic balance. No matter what comes along to upset the balance, the body knows its own nature, knows what ideal temperature it should be and the correct chemistry it needs to maintain, and keeps referring back to that blueprint to maintain proper balance.

It is like a 747 on a transoceanic flight. The pilot knows precisely what course to be on, but in order to maintain it, he has to make adjustments every few minutes. The body is adjusting every second of every day.

Similarly, if we break a bone in our arm, nature has the intelligence and know-how to heal it. All the doctor does is put the arm in a cast so we don't interfere with the healing process.

The intelligence of the immune system purifying out foreign elements, of the broken bone mending itself, or of the body ceaselessly adapting itself to changing circumstances are all part of the magnificent intelligence inherent everywhere in nature. The purpose of Ayurveda is to keep that intelligence lively in us to the maximum degree; to attune our lives to the wisdom at the heart of nature and be guided by it, so that it can regulate our lives with the same flawless intelligence it uses to revolve the galaxies.

A New Dimension of Healing

Ayurveda adds an entirely new dimension to our understanding and experience of life. It offers more than dietary advice, exercise plans, herbal supplements, and so forth, to treat the body; more than intellectual understanding of our constitution; more than emotional release; more than music therapy, aromatherapy, and other ways of enlivening the senses.

It does all this. But it also includes the deepest level of our being, our innermost spiritual center, in its model of the complete human being and in its methodology for attaining perfect health.

The Self, as this inner dimension of our nature is called in Ayurveda, is the central point of our being, the hub of the wheel. It is the true inner center of our diversified lives. Thought, feelings, speech, action, and relationships all originate here, deep within the personality. The whole person—and the whole field of interpersonal behavior—can be spontaneously enhanced by the process of *Self-referral,* or looking within to experience the Self. This is analogous to the natural process by which all the branches, leaves, flowers, and fruit of a tree can be simultaneously nourished and enlivened by watering the root.

The Self can be directly experienced. Those who do experience it find it to be deeply peaceful, yet a reservoir of creativity, intelligence, and happiness that spills over into all phases of living.

In this book we will sometimes refer to *Maharishi* Ayur-Veda. This is to acknowledge the contributions of Maharishi Mahesh Yogi, known throughout the world as the founder of the Transcendental Meditation program. For decades the Maharishi has actively promoted a worldwide revival of Ayurveda, in a modern scientific framework. The organizations founded by him, which teach Ayurveda and provide treatments employing Ayurvedic techniques, always use the name, Maharishi Ayur-Veda.

Maharishi's contributions are especially noteworthy with reference to the importance of *consciousness*—the experience of the Self and the process of Self-referral—as a key element in health and healing. This element has always been part of Ayurveda. Charaka, one of the great "founding fathers" of Ayurvedic medicine, said that "the physician who does not reach the inner self of the patient by the light of his knowledge will not be able to properly treat the disease." Yet this approach has long been given a secondary place, far behind approaches dealing primarily with physical health.

The importance of the consciousness approach is that it strengthens from a deeper level than do herbs, exercises, or any other sort of treatment. If you can heal from the source, you can, in one stroke, heal the whole as well as any and all parts. This is holistic medicine at its best.

Prevention—Your Key to Long-Term Good Health

Ayurveda holds that specific disease conditions are symptoms of an underlying imbalance. It does not neglect relief of these symptoms, but its main focus is on the big picture: to restore balance and to help you create such a healthy lifestyle that the imbalance won't occur again.

That is why Ayurveda doesn't emphasize the "attack the symptoms" approach so familiar in Western medicine. (A cold medication, for example, dries up your sinuses and stops some of the symptoms, but it doesn't really get rid of the cold.) Ayurveda, by contrast, aims to purify and strengthen the whole person and attune our life to natural rhythms and natural laws so that problems don't arise. This preventive approach requires putting a little time and attention on your health, but it is very much worth it: It's highly cost-effective in the long run, saving you from doctor bills, medicines with their potential negative side effects, and all the discomforts and possibly serious consequences of illness.

From this perspective, you will find suggestions in this book that might seem unusual to you. If you have digestive problems, rather than be told to "take this herb to make you feel better," I might recommend that you eat your largest meal at noon, when the "digestive fire" in the body is strongest. Of course, you will also find specific remedies to help you deal immediately with an irritating or painful condition, but I would not be true to the heart and essence of Ayurveda if I didn't give you the steps to bring about lasting healing and a state of perfect balance.

Living in health and balance is the key to a long life free from disease.

Choose to Be Healthy

Perhaps the most important lesson Ayurveda has to teach is that our health is not ultimately in the hands of doctors; it is up to us. Every day of our lives, every hour of every day, we can—and do—choose either health or illness.

If, for example, we eat fresh, natural foods and get some appropriate exercise, if we rest enough, stay on a reasonable routine, and surround ourselves with upbeat people and uplifting stimuli, we are choosing health and are actively *creating* health. If we eat badly and don't get proper exercise, if we live erratically, indulge in negative emotions, and burn ourselves out with overwork and stress, we are creating the fertile ground for illness. It's really that simple.

When we choose wisely, Nature rewards us with health and happiness. When we persistently choose unwisely, Nature, in her wisdom, eventually sets us straight: She makes us sick and gives us a chance to rest and rethink our choices.

The purpose of this book is to give you all the knowledge you need in order to make the right choices—for you. It is for people who want to take an active, intelligent, informed part in their own health maintenance and health creation.

You Are Unique

You are a unique person, with unique needs. The health guidelines that are right for you may be inappropriate for someone else. And yet modern Western medicine generally treats everyone alike. We are all given the same recommendations for nutrition, for example, cereal and a glass of orange juice for breakfast, and the same standard prescription for exercise. But quite a few people get gas or heartburn from orange juice, and aerobic exercise several times a week—the usual prescription these days—would be quite unnecessary, even stressful or dangerous, for many of us.

According to Ayurveda, because we each have a unique constitution, our health prescription must be unique to us. This means that in order to be healthy, you need to eat certain foods that are beneficial for your body type and stay away from others. Your exercise program must be personally suitable as well. Your constitution determines very much about you—your body, your personality, even how you relate to other people. Understanding it lets you know what you need in order to be healthy.

If you needed to work on your car's electrical system, a standard all-purpose owner's manual labeled "Car" would not be of much value. You would need one that told you what to do specifically for your Toyota or your Mercedes, your Ford or your Cadillac. Western medicine tends to provide a generic health manual, supposedly valid for all models. Fortunately, Ayurveda provides an owner's manual more specifically for you. Whatever your body type, the guidelines in this book can help you maintain balance, vitality, and joy of living.

In the next chapter, and continuing throughout the book, I will paint a detailed picture of these constitutional types, show you how to know what yours is, and give you specific lifestyle guidelines— diet, exercise, daily routine, and more—for your unique type. If you follow these guidelines, you can create balance and vitality in your mind and body, improve your relationships dramatically, and lead a long, fully healthy life.

HAPTER 2

YOUR BODY TYPE
MASTER KEY TO HEALTH

Have you ever wondered why some people can eat all they want and still remain thin, while others seem to put on weight if they just *look* at food?

Have you noticed that some people can go out in the cold without a coat and feel completely comfortable, while others have cold hands and feet even on warm, sunny days?

Do you know the reason some people have a strong sex drive, while others seem completely comfortable with infrequent sex?

The answers to these questions are contained in the ancient Ayurvedic system of classifying individuals according to their body type or constitution.*

The unique constellation of elements that makes up your body type is vitally important. According to Ayurveda, each type requires a diet, exercise program, and lifestyle specifically tailored for that type. To be healthy, you must know who you are!

This is because the food you eat, how much or what kind of exercise you do, the seasons, the weather, even the time of day all

---

*It would be more accurate to say *mind-body* type rather than just body type, since it takes into consideration mental, emotional, and spiritual as well as physical tendencies and characteristics. But for the sake of simplicity, I'm going to refer to "body types" or "constitutional types" in this book.

have different effects on different people, *according to their body type.*

Once you know your type you can make intelligent choices about what you can eat and what you can't, how much and what type of exercise is best for you, and so on. You will understand what kinds of situations tend to upset you and what you can do about them. You will be able to organize your life and create a daily routine that will keep you in perfect mental and physical balance.

Knowledge of body types is also an important key for relationships, as you'll find out later in the book. Knowing your partner's body type can foster mutual understanding and appreciation and minimize conflicts.

If you are a parent, knowledge of your child's constitutional type will enable you to provide the right environment and guidance for his or her health and happiness. Simple things, such as preparing food appropriate for your child's constitution or suggesting the most beneficial games and sports, can make all the difference between a happy, balanced, childhood and a troubled one leading to more problems later.

So this is an important, crucial chapter. In the first few pages you will learn some basic principles behind the classification of body types, and I'll give you examples to familiarize you with each of the main types. Then I'll ask you a few questions to help you determine the nature of your own constitution.

This is knowledge you MUST have in order to make use of all the hundreds of practical suggestions in the chapters that follow. I know you are eager to get on to those suggestions, but please be patient and go through this chapter carefully. You may also want to return to it later, to clarify or remind yourself of some of these principles.

Three Building Blocks of Man and Nature

According to classical Ayurveda, everything in nature is made up of five elements: space, air, fire, water, and earth. These five elements combine to form three basic qualities or *doshas,* called *Vata, Pitta,* and *Kapha:*

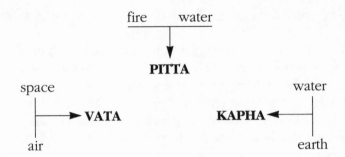

Ayurveda characterizes all things in nature according to their relative proportions of Vata, Pitta, and Kapha. These three qualities are present everywhere—in minerals, plants, and animals, as well as in our bodies.

> *VATA* (pronounced vah'tuh) refers to movement and flow. In our bodies, Vata governs the functioning of the nervous system and the movement within the other bodily systems, such as respiration, intestinal peristalsis, menstruation, excretion, etc.
>
> *PITTA* (pit'tuh) refers to digestion and metabolism. It governs our processes of digestion and absorption of nutrients.
>
> *KAPHA* (kah'fuh) is the principle of structure, fluidity, and cohesiveness. In our bodies Kapha governs our physical structure and fluid balance.

We need all three of these doshas in order to maintain life. Vata allows us to breathe and is the principle behind the flow of blood through our veins and the movement of food through the digestive tract. Nerves send their swift messages under the influence of Vata. We need Pitta to process (metabolize) food, air, and water. Kapha gives us our structure, holding together not just cells but also our muscles, fat, and bones.

The Constitutional Types

Ayurveda classifies people into constitutional types according to the doshas that predominate in their makeup. A few people may be characterized by a single dosha, but most of us are combinations of two or more. We can be:

Vata

Pitta

Kapha

Vata-Pitta

Pitta-Vata

Vata-Kapha

Kapha-Vata

Pitta-Kapha

Kapha-Pitta

Vata-Pitta-Kapha

You will notice that I mention both Vata-Pitta and Pitta-Vata, Vata-Kapha and Kapha-Vata, Pitta-Kapha and Kapha-Pitta. A Vata-Pitta is a person whose body type is predominantly Vata and secondarily Pitta; a Pitta-Vata is the reverse, primarily Pitta, secondarily Vata. The same goes for the other pairs.

It's beyond the scope of this book to go into detail about the characteristics of each of the ten constitutional types. The following explanations of the three basic body types, combined with the body type test at the end of the chapter, will give you plenty of information to understand your own constitution. I'm sure you'll also begin to see characteristics of your friends, co-workers, and family members in these descriptions.

Valerie:* A typical vata

Valerie is an artist and art teacher at a metropolitan university. A lively and entertaining speaker, she keeps her students engaged with her enthusiasm and quick wit. She is highly creative but has a hard time working consistently and finishing projects she starts.

In fact, consistency in any area of her life is not her forte. Her schedule—when she gets up, when she eats her meals, when she goes to bed—varies from day to day. Often, she'll skip a meal, simply forgetting about it. When she's enthusiastic about a person, a book, or a painting she's working on, she may stay up till the early hours of morning. Even her relationships tend to lack consistency;

---

*In this book the names, places, and circumstances of individuals referred to in the case histories have been modified to protect confidentiality.

CHARACTERISTICS OF VATA TYPES

Here are some of the common characteristics of people who have a predominantly Vata body type. In reading these, it may help to remember that Vata is composed of the space and air elements (corresponding to our senses of hearing and touch) and that characteristic qualities of Vata include dry, mobile, cold, light, changeable, subtle, rough, and quick.

- Creativity, mental quickness
- Highly imaginative
- Quick to learn and grasp new knowledge, but also quick to forget
- Sexually easily excitable but quickly satiated
- Slenderness; lightest of the three body types
- Talk and walk quickly
- Tendency toward cold hands and feet, discomfort in cold climates
- Excitable, lively, fun personality
- Changeable moods
- Irregular daily routine
- Variable appetite and digestive efficiency
- High energy in short bursts; tendency to tire easily and to overexert
- Full of joy and enthusiasm when in balance
- Respond to stress with fear, worry, and anxiety, especially when out of balance
- Tendency to act on impulse
- Often have racing, disjointed thoughts
- Generally have dry skin and dry hair and don't perspire much
- Typical health problems include headaches, hypertension, dry coughs, sore throats, earaches, anxiety, irregular heart rhythms, muscle spasms, lower back pain, constipation, abdominal gas, diarrhea, nervous stomach, menstrual cramps, premature ejaculation and other sexual dysfunctions, arthritis. Most neurological disorders are related to Vata imbalance.

Health Tip: The most important thing for Vatas to accomplish—and often the most difficult—is to maintain regular habits, that is, to eat and sleep at regular times. When Vata is out of balance this may feel almost impossible, but an effort to establish a regular routine is very important for all people with a Vata body type.

Valerie has married twice and moved restlessly through a number of relationships in between.

When Valerie is happy and in balance, she is enthusiastic and full of life. Her *joie de vivre* can be quite infectious, and she is imaginative and creative in everything—dress, home decoration, cooking—as well as in her artwork and teaching. She can be excitable, and her moods tend to shift quite rapidly. She tires pretty easily, but she'll push herself and keep going, eventually getting exhausted.

Valerie has a light, slender figure. Since childhood, she has had a hard time "putting meat on her bones"; no matter how much she eats, she remains narrow from her shoulders to her knees. Her skin is fair, but tends toward dryness, especially in winter.

She's very sensitive to her surroundings, particularly to sounds; she doesn't tolerate noise well.

When Valerie is under stress she has a tendency to become fearful and anxious. Her lively nature can turn into nonstop talking, and her charming unpredictability may suddenly seem like indecisiveness or erratic behavior. Physically, some of Valerie's recurring problems include constipation, insomnia, lower back pain, menstrual cramps, and headaches.

Peter: example of a pitta body type

Like most people with a Pitta constitution, Peter has a good-looking, strong, medium-sized build—neither too thin nor too stocky. He has reddish-blond hair, thinning somewhat early in life. His skin is fair, dotted with freckles here and there, and needs to be kept out of the sun or risk burning. His eyes have a penetrating gaze.

A basketball player in high school, now as Peter moves into middle age he is focusing on perfecting his tennis game. But reminiscent of tennis star John McEnroe, Peter's will to win and his hot temper—typical of Pitta types—sometimes leads to emotional outbursts on the court. He doesn't like to lose.

His competitive energy serves him well at work, where it has given him a leadership role and resulted in steady advancement. On the other hand, his intensity and ambition tend to make him domineering over others, who resent it. This intense quality may be playing a role in an ulcer that is developing and is surely at the root of Peter's marital problems—though his success has brought prosperity to his family, his wife does not appreciate his irritability and out-

CHARACTERISTICS OF PITTA TYPES

Here are some of the common characteristics of people who have a predominantly Pitta body type. In reading these, it may help to remember that Pitta is composed of the fire and water elements (corresponding to the senses of sight and taste) and that characteristic qualities of Pitta include hot, sharp, light, moist, slightly oily, fluid, and sour-smelling.

- Medium physique, strong, well-built
- Sharp mind, good concentration powers
- Orderly, focused
- Assertive, self-confident, and entrepreneurial at their best; aggressive, demanding, pushy when out of balance
- Competitive, enjoy challenges
- Passionate and romantic; sexually have more vigor and endurance than Vatas, but less than Kaphas
- Strong digestion, strong appetite; get irritated if they have to miss or wait for a meal
- Like to be in command
- When under stress, Pittas become irritated and angry
- Skin fair or reddish, often with freckles; sunburns easily
- Hair usually fine and straight, tending toward blond or red; typically turns gray early; tendency toward baldness or thinning hair
- Uncomfortable in sun or hot weather; heat makes them very tired
- Perspire a lot
- Others may find them stubborn, pushy, opinionated
- Good public speakers; also capable of sharp, sarcastic, cutting speech
- Generally good management and leadership ability, but can become authoritarian
- Like to spend money, surround themselves with beautiful objects
- Subject to temper tantrums, impatience, and anger
- Typical physical problems include rashes or inflammations of the skin, acne, boils, skin cancer, ulcers, heartburn, acid stomach, hot sensations in the stomach or intestines, insomnia, bloodshot or burning eyes and other vision problems, anemia, jaundice.

Health Tip: *Pitta constitutions will be upset by alcohol and cigarettes, as well as by overwork, overexertion, and overheating. When out of balance, they are susceptible to feeling such negative emotions as hostility, hatred, intolerance, and jealousy. Therefore it is very important for Pittas to keep cool (literally and figuratively) and to lead a pure and moderate lifestyle.*

bursts of anger, nor the "workaholic" nature that regularly keeps him late at the office.

Peter has a strong digestion and strong appetite; he can be ravenously hungry and can become quite upset if he has to wait for a meal. He can eat a lot and almost anything, but certain "hot" foods are beginning to create heartburn and are also contributing to the ulcer.

Like most people with a Pitta personality, Peter is strong-minded, enterprising, bold, and outspoken. He has a sharp intellect and strong powers of concentration. An excellent public speaker, his precise, articulate speech reflects his orderly mind.

Characteristically, he tends to create order in his environment, but like many Pittas, he tends to order *people* around, too; Pittas usually feel they are meant to be in charge of every situation.

Warm, impassioned, focused, successful when he is balanced and at his best, Peter can become impatient, authoritarian, and "hot under the collar" when out of balance.

Karen: A kapha body type

From the time she was a little girl, Karen was unusually affectionate and warm. Patient, nonjudgmental, forgiving, she was the one people came to in high school and college when they needed a friend. She was always a good listener, always compassionate. These qualities helped make her an outstanding mother and a supportive wife and have helped her as a therapist, the career she took up when her children were in school.

Like most people with a Kapha constitution, Karen has a relatively large build, with big bones. Her full, curvaceous figure and calm, self-contained disposition give her an "Earth Mother" image. She has thick hair and smooth, pale skin, with large, dark, "liquid" eyes.

Like most Kaphas, Karen has excellent resistance to disease and has enjoyed good health all her life.

She has always been capable of hard physical work and often joked that she should have been a farmer. Physical fatigue is almost unknown to Kaphas when they are in balance. Yet they also need the most sleep. Karen feels she has to have nine hours or she doesn't function well.

The calm, relaxed, Kapha steadiness that Karen expresses when she is in balance is just a step away from stagnation and inertia, which she must always guard against. She needs to push herself to get plenty of exercise and stimulation, or she will naturally incline toward the known, the easy, the status quo.

As Vatas are very sensitive to sound and Pittas to visual stimuli and light, Kaphas are oriented around taste and smell. Food is very important to them. Karen is one of many Kapha types who has a tendency to use food for emotional comfort. She can easily put excess weight on her large frame, and her slow metabolism and tendency toward complacency make it difficult to take it off.

Kaphas are the world's natural couch potatoes. Between her family and her career Karen doesn't have time to sink into that kind of lethargy for long. But if she is ever under stress or gets out of balance, she will be a good candidate for depression, a common Kapha problem.

Kaphas also have a tendency toward possessiveness, a trait Karen exhibits in a mild way, as she has a hard time throwing things away.

"Slow and steady"—that goes a long way in describing Karen. She moves slowly, eats slowly, digests slowly, talks slowly, and makes decisions slowly. She gets started slowly in the morning, likes to lie in bed awhile before getting up, and may need a cup of coffee to get rolling. She also learns slowly, but once she learns something, she rarely forgets, as she has an excellent memory.

As for the "steady" part—she is a true-blue, faithful friend and wife. Her steadfastness and even-tempered nature provide a feeling of security. Where a Pitta type will be outspoken and combative, Karen, like most Kaphas, is a peacemaker and harmonizer.

Another of the keynotes of Kapha is sweetness, and Karen is a perfect example. Her voice is soft and low-pitched, and people know her for her kind, tolerant disposition. However, Karen also shares the Kapha love for *eating* sweets, which can too easily lead to weight gain.

As you read through the preceding examples, you probably felt, "I have many of the qualities of one type, but I have some qualities of the other types, too." This is an accurate observation. These examples were of pure Vata, Pitta, and Kapha types, but in real life, hardly anybody is a pure type; most of us are combinations in which one type predominates and the other two are present in lesser degrees.

CHARACTERISTICS OF KAPHA TYPES

Here are some of the common characteristics of people who have a predominantly Kapha body type. In reading these, it may help to remember that Kapha is composed of the earth and water elements (corresponding to smell and taste) and that characteristic qualities of Kapha include heavy, cold, oily, sweet, steady, slow, soft, sticky, dull, smooth.

- Easygoing, relaxed, slow-paced
- Affectionate and loving
- Forgiving, compassionate, nonjudgmental nature
- Stable and reliable; faithful
- Physically strong and with a sturdy, heavier build
- Have the most energy of all constitutions, but it is steady and enduring, not explosive
- Slow moving and graceful
- Slow speech, reflecting a deliberate thought process
- Slower to learn, but never forgets; outstanding long-term memory
- Soft hair and skin; tendency to have large "soft" eyes and a low, soft voice
- Tend toward being overweight; may also suffer from sluggish digestion
- Prone to heavy, oppressive depressions
- More self-sufficient, need less outward stimulation than do the other types
- A mild, gentle, and essentially undemanding approach to life
- Sexually Kaphas are the slowest to be aroused, but they also have the most endurance
- Excellent health, strong resistance to disease
- Slow to anger; strive to maintain harmony and peace in their surroundings
- Not easily upset and can be a point of stability for others
- Tend to be possessive and hold on to things, people, money; good savers
- Don't like cold, damp weather
- Physical problems include colds and congestion, sinus headaches, respiratory problems including asthma and wheezing, hay fever, allergies, and atherosclerosis (hardening of the arteries).

Health Tip: *Prone to lethargy, sluggishness, depression, and overweight, Kaphas need activity and stimulation. Daily exercise is more important for them than for any other type. Getting out of the house and actively seeking new experiences is also valuable.*

The Principle of Balance— Key to Total Health

A healthy person is one whose doshas are balanced. That is, the right proportion of Vata, Pitta, and Kapha is present *for that individual.*

To maintain strength and balance, a person with a light, fast-paced Vata constitution requires a diet consisting of heavier and oilier foods and only mild exercise. A Kapha person needs the opposite: a lighter, drier diet and more intensive exercise to stay in top mental and physical shape.

People with a Vata nature, having the qualities of dryness and coldness, need to avoid getting cold or being exposed to too much wind. They may feel uncomfortable in excessively dry climates; they will feel better if they eat foods that are warm and moist, such as soups. Pittas, whose characteristic qualities include heat and moisture, thrive in cool, dry climates; hot, humid summers can be torture to them. They feel better when they avoid spicy foods.

From this you can see that a fundamental principle of Ayurveda is that factors that *increase* Vata will tend to throw Vata constitutions out of balance (but may be helpful for Pittas or Kaphas); factors that reduce or *pacify* Vata will help Vatas maintain or restore mental, emotional, and physical balance. The same principle applies to Pittas and Kaphas. Thus I will frequently use the terms *Vata* (or *Pitta* or *Kapha*) *increasing or aggravating,* and *Vata* (or *Pitta* or *Kapha*) *balancing or pacifying* when referring to foods, herbs, exercises, and so on, that promote imbalance or balance.

Body Types: Your Master Key to Health

Now you know why body types are so important. Knowing your type is a prerequisite to putting the principles and techniques of Ayurveda into practice. More than that, it is a master key to perfect health, for once you know what makes you tick, you can easily learn how to regulate your life to maintain maximum balance. All the recommendations in the book—for diet, exercise, and so on—are directed toward a particular psycho-physiological or mind-body makeup. What is good for Vatas is not necessarily what is good for Pittas or Kaphas. You need to know what is good for *you*.

Therefore, the first step in making this program work for you is to determine the nature of your constitution.

Discover Your Constitutional Type

Use the following questionnaire to ascertain your body type. This questionnaire, however, can give you only a general idea. In order to fully understand your constitution it's important to get a complete evaluation from a physician or other health professional trained in Ayurveda.

Mind-Body Type Test

Instructions: Circle the number that applies best to each statement. Remember: This is for you to gain better self-understanding, not to enhance your self-image. In other words, be as truthful as you can. To help you get an accurate picture of yourself, you may wish to have a friend, spouse, or someone who knows you well see if they agree with your answers.

	Doesn't Apply		*Applies Somewhat*			*Applies Most*
1. I have difficulty falling asleep, or have light, interrupted sleep.	0	1	2	3	4	5	6
2. I perform activity quickly.	0	1	2	3	4	5	6
3. I'm generally lively and enthusiastic about life.	0	1	2	3	4	5	6
4. I prefer warm weather to cool weather; I don't like cold weather.	0	1	2	3	4	5	6
5. I tend to have gas and/or constipation.	0	1	2	3	4	5	6
6. My skin is dry, especially in the winter.	0	1	2	3	4	5	6
7. I have a thin physique; I don't put on weight easily.	0	1	2	3	4	5	6
8. I'm basically a positive, optimistic person.	0	1	2	3	4	5	6

9. I usually walk quickly.	0	1	2	3	4	5	6
10. I often have a hard time making decisions.	0	1	2	3	4	5	6
11. My feet and hands get cold easily.	0	1	2	3	4	5	6
12. I thrive on change; I love new things, people, and places.	0	1	2	3	4	5	6
13. I have always learned quickly, but I also forget easily.	0	1	2	3	4	5	6
14. When I'm under stress, I tend to become anxious or worried.	0	1	2	3	4	5	6
15. I'm a good communicator, but I can talk quite a lot.	0	1	2	3	4	5	6
16. My eating and sleeping habits tend to be irregular or erratic if I don't have to be on a regular routine.	0	1	2	3	4	5	6
17. I have an active, creative mind, but it tends to be restless.	0	1	2	3	4	5	6
18. I tend to tire easily and some-times burn out from overexertion.	0	1	2	3	4	5	6
19. I am flexible and can easily change directions, maybe too easily.	0	1	2	3	4	5	6
20. My moods change rapidly.	0	1	2	3	4	5	6

After you have completed these first 20 statements, add together all the numbers you have circled. This will give your total score for Vata constitutional type tendencies.

TOTAL VATA SCORE *67*

	Doesn't Apply	Applies Somewhat	Applies Most
1. I have moles, freckles, or acne problems.	0 1 2	3 4	5 6
2. I can eat a lot; my appetite is good and my digestion is strong.	0 1 2	3 4	5 6
3. My hair is thin and silky; and/or			

I have an early appearance of baldness or graying; and/or my hair is blond, sandy, or red.   0   1   2   3   4   5   6

4. I prefer cold foods and drinks.   0   1   2   3   4   5   6

5. I dislike being out in the sun for a long time.   0   1   2   3   4   5   6

6. I like to be in charge and do things my way.   0   1   2   3   4   5   6

7. I prefer cool weather to hot weather; I feel uncomfortable or tired in the heat.   0   1   2   3   4   5   6

8. I have a sharp intellect.   0   1   2   3   4   5   6

9. I perspire easily.   0   1   2   3   4   5   6

10. I am confident and enjoy challenges.   0   1   2   3   4   5   6

11. I become uncomfortable if I have to miss a meal or get to it late.   0   1   2   3   4   5   6

12. I tend to be orderly and perfectionistic.   0   1   2   3   4   5   6

13. Under stress, I tend to lose my temper or feel irritated.   0   1   2   3   4   5   6

14. I tend to stick to my own ideas and views; I can be quite stubborn.   0   1   2   3   4   5   6

15. I become impatient when others are slow or disorganized.   0   1   2   3   4   5   6

16. When I want something, I go for it aggressively.   0   1   2   3   4   5   6

17. I have a medium build with a well developed physique (not thin, not stout).   0   1   2   3   4   5   6

18. At my worst, my aggressiveness can make me dominating or manipulative.   0   1   2   3   4   5   6

19. I have a warm, friendly, outgoing nature.   0   1   2   3   4   5   6

20. But I also can become irritable and angry quite easily.   0   1   2   3   4   5   6

Now add the numbers you just circled in the same way you did for your Vata score. The sum of the numbers you circled for these 20 statements gives you your Pitta constitutional type score.

TOTAL PITTA SCORE ___73___

	Doesn't Apply		Applies Somewhat			Applies Most	
1. I eat slowly and tend to do most things slowly and methodically.	0	1	2	3	4	5	6
2. I care a lot about other people's feelings and try to keep things peaceful and harmonious.	0	1	2	3	4	5	6
3. I am generally tolerant, patient, and slow to get irritated.	0	1	2	3	4	5	6
4. I rarely get sick.	0	1	2	3	4	5	6
5. When I do get sick, I tend to have a runny nose or excess phlegm, congestion, asthma, sinus problems, or allergies.	0	1	2	3	4	5	6
6. I usually have a deep sleep that tends to last eight hours or more.	0	1	2	3	4	5	6
7. I'm a little slow at learning new things.	0	1	2	3	4	5	6
8. My skin is naturally soft, smooth, and on the oily side.	0	1	2	3	4	5	6
9. I can easily skip a meal without discomfort; I don't get upset if a meal is delayed.	0	1	2	3	4	5	6
10. I have a good long-term memory; once I have learned facts, names, etc., I remember them for a long time.	0	1	2	3	4	5	6
11. I have a peaceful, happy disposition that is hard to disturb.	0	1	2	3	4	5	6
12. I don't have a huge appetite, but I tend to put on weight easily anyway; I've always tended to be heavy.	0	1	2	3	4	5	6

13. My least favorite weather is cool
and damp.   0   1   2   3   4   5   <u>6</u>

14. My walk is slow and relaxed.   0   1   2   3   4   <u>5</u>   6

15. I have a high level of physical
strength and stamina.   0   <u>1</u>   2   3   4   5   6

16. I tend to be a somewhat passive,
receptive person. I am not an
aggressive type.   0   1   2   <u>3</u>   4   5   6

17. I am loyal, faithful, and devoted.   0   1   2   3   4   5   <u>6</u>

18. I have a romantic, sentimental
streak. I tend to get attached to
things and people and have a
hard time letting go.   0   1   <u>2</u>   3   4   5   6

19. I can be quite lethargic and
apathetic and even depressed.   0   1   2   3   4   <u>5</u>   6

20. I am basically a patient, loving,
nurturing, supportive person.   0   1   2   3   4   <u>5</u>   6

Again, tally the numbers you circled in these statements to get your total Kapha score.

TOTAL KAPHA SCORE   <u>71</u>

Now, compare your three scores for Vata, Pitta, and Kapha. Whichever of the three is highest is your predominant dosha. The second highest is the second strongest dosha, and the lowest is your least dominant dosha.

If the highest score is much higher than either of the other two—twice as big, for example—you may qualify as a "pure" personality type. For example, if you scored "94" for Vata, "36" for Pitta, and "25" for Kapha, you might well be a Vata type personality. Usually, though, people are a mixture of two or three doshas. If, for example, you scored "75" for Vata, "61" for Pitta, and "33" for Kapha, you're more likely a Vata-Pitta type.

Again, a questionnaire can give you only a rough approximation of your constitution. To be certain, I strongly recommend a consultation with an Ayurvedic physician. (See Appendix B.)

However, there is a way that you can verify the questionnaire and at the same time learn a marvelous technique to monitor your health, and that is to gain the skill of pulse diagnosis.

Pulse Diagnosis: A Window into Your Inner Functioning

One of the ways the Ayurvedic physician uses to determine your body type and your current condition is to take your pulse. To the skilled pulse diagnostician, taking the pulse is not merely counting the beats, but a way of looking closely into the functioning of the entire system. The underlying constitutional type is immediately evident, and also the entire state of the body, including the balance of the doshas, the health of the various organs, minor problems that may lead to illness later on, etc.

This ancient method of diagnosis could be likened to a human, non-technological CAT scan or MRI scan, because an expert in pulse diagnosis is able, by feeling the impulses as they pass through the pulse, to detect any imbalances in the entire psychology and physiology. For our purposes now, all we want to learn is how to determine the constitutional type. This is how you do it:

• Hold the palm of one hand facing up. Put your other hand, also facing up, *underneath* that wrist. (Traditionally, men reach under with the left hand and feel the right pulse, women feel the left pulse with the right hand.)

• Now locate the small rounded bone on your top wrist, just below the base of the thumb. Place your fingers just beyond the bone so that the first finger comes right below the bone. In that position, you will be able to feel the throbbing of the radial pulse.

• Now line up the first three fingers. If you press down fairly firmly and pay close attention, you will feel slightly different pulsations under each finger. Your index finger will be detecting the Vata pulse, your middle finger the Pitta pulse, and your ring finger the Kapha pulse. (You may have to press just a little harder to pick up the Kapha pulse, particularly if you have little Kapha in your constitution. The reason is that the radial artery moves deeper under the flesh as it moves up the arm away from the wrist.)

• You will notice that there is (1) an unequal strength in each pulse, and (2) a slightly different quality to each. Traditionally, it is said that the Vata pulse is like a snake, quick, irregular, and slithery. The Pitta pulse is more regular, more forceful and jumpy, likened to the leaping of a frog. The Kapha pulse will be slower and steadier, said to be like the graceful gliding of a swan.

• You can tell your body type by the relative strength of the pulse under the three fingers.

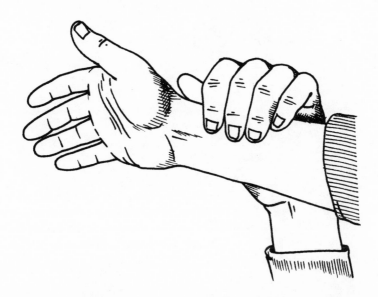

Please remember that the art of accurate pulse diagnosis requires not only sensitivity, but training, careful, quiet attention, and lots of practice. You may have a knack for it and pick up the basics right away, but don't be discouraged if you're not immediately successful. In the training of an Ayurvedic physician, the student first practices for a long time on himself, then is expected to do as many as 100 readings a day on others for a long time before he is competent to make medical diagnoses.

Thank you for your patience in learning a few of the fundamental principles of Ayurvedic natural medicine, and taking the time to determine your constitutional type. Now you are about to embark on the practical aspects of this wonderful system of natural healing!

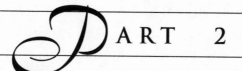

PART 2

SIX KEYS
TO PERFECT
HEALTH

CHAPTER 3

EAT RIGHT FOR YOUR BODY TYPE

You may find it hard to believe, but when many doctors were in medical school, they had as little as one or two lectures allotted to the study of nutrition, and that's often still the case today! And yet everyone knows from experience that diet and nutrition profoundly influence our moods and behavior as well as our physical health.

Food is one of the most common subjects patients bring up when they come in to see their doctors. Certain foods seem to make them tired, they say, or irritable; others affect their digestion, seem to give them insomnia, or upset their normal sleep. Since most physicians are not trained in the area of nutrition, they usually pay little attention to these observations, though they might contain an important clue to their patient's health.

Frank and Susie went out for a pizza. It tasted great to both of them, but afterward, Frank felt congested, dull-minded, and had such a bad stomach ache he vowed never to eat pizza again. Susie felt just fine. Why? Because the pizza was appropriate for her constitutional type. Being a Pitta-Vata with a strong "digestive fire," she had no problem digesting the wheat and cheese. But it was poison for Frank, whose Kapha constitution immediately got plugged up and made him uncomfortable.

Modern medical science is finally beginning to acknowledge that the food we eat has a direct and vital effect upon our health.

35

The National Cancer Institute and American Heart Association, for example, have both indicated that a diet low in fiber and high in meat is correlated with a higher incidence of colon cancer, heart disease, and stroke. The American Cancer Society has stated that as many as 35 percent of the 900,000 new cases of cancer each year in the United States could be prevented simply by following proper dietary recommendations.

For thousands of years, Ayurveda has provided a complete and systematic understanding about the effects of food upon our mental and physical functioning. In this chapter you will learn basic Ayurvedic dietary principles, including the system for classifying foods. You will discover which foods are good for your constitution, which ones you should avoid, and which ones are all right under certain circumstances.

Digestion is also considered to be very important. It's not only *what* we eat that matters; *how* we eat and how well our system processes the food is also crucial. Later, I'm going to devote an entire chapter (10) to tips on how to eat and how to strengthen your digestion in order to gain maximum nutritional benefit from the food you eat.

The dietary recommendations in this chapter can be used

1. as *preventive medicine* to keep a healthy person healthy, or
2. *for healing and restoring balance* if some particular illness or imbalance comes up. Then a particular type of diet, along with herbal preparations, can be emphasized in order to bring the system back to normal.

How You Can Use Food to Create Balance

In every item of creation there is a specific balance of Vata, Pitta, and Kapha. Ayurveda has classified all plants, minerals, and animals according to their unique proportion of these three doshas. This system tells us what food should be eaten by what person for what purpose. For example, cooling food is good for a hot person in the summer, warm food for a cold person in the winter, drying food for a congested person, strengthening food for a weak person, and so on.

HOW TO USE THE PRINCIPLE OF SIMILARITIES AND DIFFERENCES TO RESTORE BALANCE

Similarities: When there is an excess of any quality (dosha) in the body, taking in anything (food, herb, mineral, etc.) that has *similar* properties will cause that quality to *increase*. For example, when there is an excess of Vata, eating Vata-increasing foods, taking Vata-increasing herbs, etc., will make the Vata aggravation worse.

Differences: When there is an excess of any quality (dosha) in the body, taking in anything (food, herb, mineral, etc.) that is *opposite* to the excess in the body will cause the imbalance to *decrease*. For example, if there is excess Kapha, eating Kapha-pacifying foods, taking Kapha-pacifying herbs, etc., will help to alleviate the imbalance.

When there's an excess of one quality, giving the opposite has a balancing effect. If there's too much heat (Pitta) in the mind/body system, resulting perhaps in excess anger, or heartburn, then taking some foods that have a cooling property will pacify the Pitta and help bring the system into balance. Some effective options would include a glass of cool water, an apple, a handful of grapes, a dish of ice cream, or a couple of spoonfuls of *ghee* (clarified butter) in a cup of warm milk.

Ruth, a 25-year-old woman, went to see her Ayurvedic physician suffering from a bad rash on both arms, with severe itching. She also felt a great deal of anger at her boyfriend, who had recently left her for another woman. She didn't connect the two symptoms, but when her doctor felt her pulse, he found that her Pitta was quite aggravated. The treatment recommended for Ruth consisted of a combination of three Ayurvedic herbs, Indian asparagus (*shatavari*), licorice root, and aloe vera, all used for pacifying Pitta. Within two days the rash was completely gone and the associated anger was giving way to understanding and acceptance of her situation. The supportive, empathic counseling her physician gave her seemed to work much better *after* the Pitta was balanced with the help of the herbs.

Each person has a unique proportion of Vata, Pitta, and Kapha in his or her constitution. Foods should be eaten that help to maintain balance in that particular physiology. Someone with a Vata constitution, which is by nature cold and dry, should emphasize foods that are opposite to these qualities. Some good choices would be

HOW THE SEASONS AFFECT THE DOSHAS

Vata increases in autumn and winter
(approximately October–February)
Kapha increases in spring
(approximately March–May)
Pitta increases in summer
(approximately June–September)

warm and moist foods such as soups, rice with a little butter, and juicy cooked vegetables such as zucchini.

The seasons also profoundly influence our mind and body by bringing out or increasing the dosha related to that season. Thus the seasons also need to be taken into consideration when deciding what to eat. Summer increases Pitta, spring increases Kapha, and autumn and winter increase Vata. (We will discuss this at length in Chapter 6.)

This becomes a little more interesting for people with two dominant doshas. For example, a person with a Vata-Pitta constitution will find Vata tending to increase during the fall season and Pitta increasing during the summer season. This means that during the fall, he or she might be more prone to develop anxiety, worry, muscle tension, insomnia, constipation, and difficulty concentrating ("spaciness"). During the summer, this same person might be prone to experience temper outbursts, irritability, skin rashes, and acid stomach or reflux esophagitis. Therefore, a Vata-pacifying diet during the fall season and a Pitta-pacifying diet during the summer season is effective preventive medicine for that person. (Please refer to the Diet Charts beginning on page 43.)

What should this Vata-Pitta person do during the spring season, when Kapha tends to increase? Although the question is more crucial for people with Kapha constitutions, even a Vata-Pitta should be careful not to increase or aggravate Kapha during the spring season, when colds and congestion easily arise. Therefore, a combination diet is recommended. In the early part of spring, when the weather is still cold, a diet that combines elements of the Vata and Kapha pacifying diets would be best; toward the end of spring, when the weather becomes warmer, a diet combining Kapha and Pitta pacifying foods will be most helpful for maintaining mental, emotional, and physical well-being.

Important: If this all seems pretty abstract right now, don't worry—soon you'll know exactly what foods go with each diet, and it will all start to make sense.

A Case of Chronic Fatigue Naturally Healed

Joan was suffering from Chronic Fatigue Syndrome, a condition characterized by extreme tiredness, low motivation, depression, and poor immunity. After several "totally frustrating" treatment suggestions from allopathically-oriented physicians, Joan consulted an Ayurvedic doctor. The fact that it was Kapha season, along with some outward signs of Kapha imbalance including overweight and sinus congestion, led the doctor to believe that Joan was suffering from a Kapha-aggravated disorder. Pulse diagnosis confirmed that this supposition was correct.

Joan was prescribed several natural, Kapha-pacifying treatments, such as gradually working toward a vigorous exercise program, steam baths, a special Ayurvedic drying massage,* a Kapha-reducing herbal mixture, as well as a Kapha-pacifying diet. She was also prescribed one of the Ayurvedic stress-management techniques, Transcendental Meditation (see Chapter 4) to increase her energy and mental clarity.

The treatment had a dramatic effect on Joan's symptoms. Within a few weeks, without medications, she was experiencing significantly more energy and vitality and was able to function at a much higher level, both at home and at her job.

Balance Your Diet with the Six Tastes

Trying to eat well according to Western nutrition can be quite complicated. To do it thoroughly, you would have to check out the chemical makeup—the vitamin, mineral, protein, and carbohydrate contents—of each item of food. Ayurveda has a far simpler system of determining nutritional value. According to this system, all the important nutrients that we need for life—fats, proteins, carbohy-

---

*This drying massage is called *udvartina*. You can do it at home by mixing sesame oil and chickpea flour into a paste and massaging it into the skin. Massage in the direction of venous circulation, i.e., inward toward the heart: upward motion from the hands toward the shoulders, from the feet toward the hips, etc.

drates, minerals, vitamins, and so on—are contained in a meal that consists of all six tastes.

The six tastes are sweet, sour, salty, bitter, pungent, and astringent. Here are some examples of foods with those tastes:

Sweet bread and all grains including rice, barley, wheat; milk but not all dairy products; many fruits; all meats; sugar; honey

Sour cheese, yogurt, vinegar, citrus fruits, tomatoes

Salty salt

Bitter green leafy vegetables such as spinach, bitter greens (romaine lettuce, endive), horseradish, turmeric

Pungent spicy foods and seasonings of all types, onions, radishes, garlic, pepper, ginger, cumin

Astringent beans and lentils, pomegranates, cabbage, broccoli, foods that have a drying, lip-puckering effect

Any meal that contains food items from all these six tastes will be a balanced meal. It will automatically contain all the nutrients that the system needs and will have a balancing influence on all the doshas.

Generally, our Western diet overemphasizes the sweet, sour, and salty tastes, typified by fast foods. A fast food lunch—hamburger, french fries with ketchup, and a coke—has just three tastes. The meat, bread, and coke are sweet; the fries are salty; the vinegar in the ketchup is sour.

It so happens that these three tastes all balance or reduce Vata. Vata imbalance is extremely prevalent in our society, due to all the rushing around we do and the insecurity, anxiety, and emptiness that so many people feel. These "fast foods" are appealing because, being Vata pacifying, they help assuage such feelings. But they are also difficult to digest, are oily in nature, and don't contain all the needed nutrition because they lack some of the six tastes. A diet such as this tends to produce an imbalance of Kapha, characterized by lethargy, overweight, depression, mental dullness, and greediness.

Here is a case where one imbalance (Vata) leads to further imbalance (Kapha). The way to break out of this vicious cycle is to eat a balanced diet, appropriate for one's own constitution, and to incorporate all six tastes in every main meal.

EFFECTS OF THE SIX TASTES

Each of the six tastes has specific effects, both beneficial and, if used in excess, potentially harmful.

SWEET—Increases Kapha, reduces Vata and Pitta. Nourishing and strengthening and promotes growth of all tissues, so is good for growing children, the elderly, and the weak or injured. Increases *ojas* and prolongs life. Good for hair, skin and complexion, and for healing broken bones. In excess, sweet taste promotes Kapha imbalances and disorders such as heaviness, laziness, and dullness, colds, obesity, excessive sleeping, loss of appetite, etc.

SOUR—Increases Pitta and Kapha, reduces Vata. Stimulates appetite, digestion, and elimination and helps dispel gas. Sharpens the mind and senses. Excess sour taste is weakening, causes itching and irritation, thirst, blood toxicity.

SALTY—Increases Pitta and Kapha, reduces Vata. Stimulates salivation and digestion. It works as a sedative and laxative and relieves stiffness. Excess salt can aggravate skin conditions, weaken the system, cause wrinkling of the skin and graying and falling out of hair. It promotes inflammatory skin diseases, gout, and other Pitta disorders.

PUNGENT—Increases Pitta and Vata, decreases Kapha. Stimulates appetite and improves digestion. Like salt and sour, pungent improves the taste of food. Gives mental clarity. Helps cure Kapha disorders such as obesity, sluggish digestion, excess water in the body. Improves circulation. Is germicidal, stops itching, facilitates sweating and elimination of *ama* (toxic accumulations). Too much pungent taste can cause weakness, fainting, feeling of weariness, impurities, burning sensations in the body.

BITTER—Increases Vata, decreases Pitta and Kapha. Tastes bad in itself but restores the sense of taste. Detoxifying and antibacterial, it also relieves burning, itching, and inflammatory skin conditions. Relieves thirst. Good for reducing fevers. Promotes digestion. Cleansing to the blood and helps remove ama in system. Excess bitter taste is debilitating to bodily tissues, causes weakness, emaciation, dizziness, and promotes Vata disorders.

ASTRINGENT—Increases Vata, reduces Pitta and Kapha. Drying and firming, astringent taste stops diarrhea, reduces sweating, and slows or stops bleeding. Antiinflammatory. Promotes healing. Excess astringent is weakening and causes premature aging. Its drying effect causes constipation and retention of gas. Promotes dry mouth. Promotes Vata disorders such as paralysis and spasms.

Heal Cravings and Addictions with the Six Tastes

If a person is eating primarily three of the six tastes (as, in our example, sweet, sour, and salty), he or she is not getting a full and proper amount of nutrition. As a result of this lack, cravings will tend to arise. Nutritional imbalance can thus be a cause of addictive behavior of all kinds. The mind/body system feels unsatisfied and needs *something*. If the person doesn't know what is missing, any kind of addictive behavior—not necessarily related to food—can result. On this basis people become addicted to tobacco, alcohol, drugs, sex, excitement, shopping, and so forth. Eating a balanced diet helps to maintain balanced doshas, which does much to help a person feel both physically and mentally satisfied. A satisfied soul does not have the cravings that lead to addiction.

How the Six Tastes Affect the Doshas
Here's how the six tastes influence the three doshas:

Decrease Vata	*Increase Vata*
Sweet	Pungent
Sour	Bitter
Salty	Astringent

Decrease Pitta	*Increase Pitta*
Sweet	Pungent
Bitter	Sour
Astringent	Salty

Decrease Kapha	*Increase Kapha*
Pungent	Sweet
Bitter	Sour
Astringent	Salty

Another way to see this is as follows:

Taste	*Vata*	*Pitta*	*Kapha*
Salt	↓	↑	↑
Sweet	↓	↓	↑
Sour	↓	↑	↑
Bitter	↑	↓	↓
Pungent	↑	↑	↓
Astringent	↑	↓	↓

It's very easy to use this information for both psychological and physiological balance. For example, Mary is a few days away from her monthly period. She's feeling bloated from fluid retention and is also immersed in a heavy mood of lethargy and depression. These are all Kapha symptoms. Mary has an excess of Kapha dosha in her system—quite common before the menstrual period.

By taking a look at the preceding charts, Mary can see that eating foods that are bitter, pungent, and astringent—such as salads or spicy vegetables—would help her restore balance and feel better both physically and emotionally. Eating or snacking on salty, sour, or sweet foods—which she often feels like doing because of her mood—tends to make matters worse. (The one exception is honey, which, although sweet, is very good for balancing Kapha.)

The same prescription would be useful for someone with sinus congestion and its associated feelings of mental dullness.

For a person who is feeling irritated and angry, an emphasis on foods that are bitter, sweet, or astringent—Pitta-pacifying—will be beneficial. Choice of herbs is based on the same principle. For example, drinking some jasmine, rose, or hibiscus tea (made from the petals of those flowers, which are sweet and/or astringent) would have a tendency to reduce irritability and produce a calming effect.

For a person with a Vata imbalance, such as trouble sleeping at night, some warm milk, which has a sweet taste, would have a soothing, pacifying effect that would help to induce a sound sleep. If you add a pinch of saffron, or some less expensive sweet and warming spices such as cardamom or nutmeg, the effect will be enhanced.

Dietary Recommendations to Maintain Balance of Vata, Pitta, and Kapha

Use the following charts to determine what foods are best for you. To use them, you must first know your body type (based on the questionnaire you filled out in Chapter 2 and, if possible, a diagnosis by an Ayurvedic physician).

Vata-Balancing Diet
Foods for Vata Constitutions to Favor

General Guidelines:
- The best Vata-balancing foods are warm, heavy, and oily and have sweet, sour, and salty taste.

- Vatas can eat larger quantities of food, but don't eat more than your digestion can handle.
- To balance Vata throughout the day, eat a substantial warm breakfast, preferably with cooked cereal, milk, toast, etc.
- Excellent Vata-balancing foods: warm, creamy soups; hot cereals; bread; and pasta with rich sauces such as "alfredo" (made with butter and cream).
- Warm milk is always good for balancing Vata.

GRAINS Rice (white or brown) and wheat are most Vata-balancing. Oats are acceptable if well-cooked (as in oatmeal), not dry (as in granola).

DAIRY All dairy products are good for balancing Vata. It is best to drink milk warm, and not with a full meal.

FRUIT Favor sweet fruit such as apricots, avocados, bananas, berries, coconut, cherries, fresh (not dried) figs, grapes, mangoes, melons, nectarines, papayas, sweet oranges, sweet pineapple, sweet plums.

VEGETABLES Vegetables for balancing Vata should be well-cooked. Raw salads are not recommended, but if you really like them, using a creamy or oily dressing, or accompanying with a dish of fresh cottage cheese will help balance the effect. Best vegetables for Vata are asparagus, beets, carrots, cucumbers, green beans, radishes, sweet potato, turnips. The following are also acceptable if used in moderate quantities, especially if you cook them in ghee or oil and use Vata-reducing spices (see below): broccoli, brussels sprouts, cauliflower, celery, eggplant, green leafy vegetables, peas, peppers, potatoes, tomatoes, zucchini.

BEANS Beans are not very good for Vata. Minimize their use except for tofu (made from ground soybeans), chickpeas, and pink lentils, all in moderate amounts. Mung beans are okay, especially as *dhal,* a light soup made from dried mung beans that is often served with rice in Indian cooking.

NUTS All nuts are acceptable. Almonds are especially good.

OILS All oils reduce Vata. Sesame oil is especially recommended.

SWEETENERS All sweeteners help balance Vata, though refined white sugar is not recommended.

MEAT AND FISH Chicken, turkey, and seafood are acceptable in small or moderate portions.

SPICES AND HERBS Most spices are good for Vata. Sweet and

heating herbs and spices are best, such as black pepper (in small amounts), cardamom, cinnamon, cloves, cumin, ginger, and mustard seed. Ginger is especially good for Vata digestion. Salt is okay for Vatas. You can also use allspice, anise, asafetida, basil, bay leaf, caraway, cilantro, fennel, nutmeg, oregano, sage, tarragon, and thyme.

Eat in small quantities or avoid

General Guidelines:

- Avoid all cold drinks, and cut down on foods that are cold, dry, and light.
- Minimize foods with pungent (spicy), bitter, and astringent tastes, though Indian and Mexican foods are generally okay (because they tend to be cooked in oil, which is soothing to Vata).
- Fasting and light diet are not recommended for Vata.

GRAINS Reduce your consumption of barley, buckwheat, corn, millet, and rye; avoid dry oats.

DAIRY All dairy foods are okay for Vata.

FRUIT Avoid all dried or unripe fruits. Minimize apples, pears, pomegranates, cranberries, though these are more acceptable if cooked.

VEGETABLES Avoid cabbage and bean sprouts. Many others should be minimized unless well-cooked; see the list of acceptable veggies, above.

BEANS Reduce or avoid most beans; see above.

MEAT AND FISH Avoid beef, pork, lamb.

SPICES AND HERBS Though most spices and herbs are okay, Vatas should not use them in large quantities. Minimize use of herbs and spices with bitter and astringent taste, such as coriander seed, fenugreek, parsley, turmeric.

Pitta-Balancing Diet
Foods for Pitta Constitutions to Favor

General Guidelines:

- The key to Pitta-balancing foods is: Keep it cool. Favor cool (but not ice-cold) food and drinks, especially in hot weather.
- The best tastes for balancing Pitta are sweet, bitter, and astringent.

- Salads are excellent for Pittas, especially in the summer.
- As much as possible, eat in relaxing, orderly, aesthetically pleasing surroundings.
- Although Pittas may gravitate toward meat, they thrive on a vegetarian diet better than any other body type.

GRAINS Barley, oats, wheat, and white rice (basmati is best).

DAIRY Milk, butter, and ghee (clarified butter). Ice cream is acceptable, as are egg whites.

FRUIT Sweet, ripe fruits. Avocados, cherries, coconut, grapes, mangoes, melons, pomegranates, and sweet (not sour) plums and pineapples. Oranges are okay only if sweet.

VEGETABLES Most vegetables are good for the Pitta-balancing diet. Asparagus, broccoli, brussels sprouts, cabbage, cauliflower, celery, cucumbers, green beans, leafy vegetables such as lettuce, spinach, and chard, mushrooms, okra, peas, potatoes, sprouts, sweet peppers, sweet potatoes, zucchini.

BEANS Don't favor beans in the Pitta-balancing diet. Chickpeas, kidney beans, mung beans, tofu and other soybean products are acceptable.

NUTS Most nuts don't belong on the Pitta diet. Coconut is okay, as are pumpkin seeds and sunflower seeds.

OILS Coconut, olive, soy, and sunflower.

SWEETENERS All sweeteners are all right except honey and molasses (they are heating).

MEAT AND FISH Chicken, shrimp, and turkey are acceptable in small amounts, though a vegetarian diet is recommended.

SPICES AND HERBS Spicy foods are generally too heating for Pitta, but these are acceptable: cardamom, cilantro, cinnamon, coriander, dill, fennel, mint, saffron, turmeric. Black pepper is okay in small amounts.

Eat in small quantities or avoid

General Guidelines:
- Salty, sour, spicy, and oily foods heat up the body and increase Pitta. Eat them only in moderation; avoid if Pitta is aggravated.
- Watch out for processed foods, which are full of fats and salt.

- Avoid alcoholic beverages, fermented foods, and coffee. These are particularly irritating to Pitta constitutions.

GRAINS Minimize brown rice, corn, millet, and rye.

DAIRY Avoid brick cheeses, cultured buttermilk, egg yolks, sour cream, and yogurt.

FRUITS Minimize consumption of sour fruits, such as grapefruit, sour oranges, olives, papayas, and unripe pineapples and plums. Apricots, bananas, berries, cherries, cranberries, peaches should be eaten in moderation.

VEGETABLES Avoid pungent vegetables such as onions, garlic, radishes, and hot peppers. Minimize beets, carrots, eggplant, tomatoes, and spinach.

SWEETENERS Don't use honey and molasses.

BEANS Avoid most beans, especially lentils.

NUTS Minimize all nuts and seeds, especially cashews, peanuts, and sesame seeds.

OILS Reduce almond, corn, safflower, and sesame oils.

MEAT AND FISH Avoid red meat and seafood. Lean toward a vegetarian diet.

SPICES AND HERBS Minimize your use of all pungent spices and herbs, including salt. This includes black pepper, celery seed, cloves, cumin, fenugreek, ginger, and mustard seed. Cut down on condiments such as barbecue sauce, strong salad dressings, vinegar, mustard, pickles, catsup. Completely avoid chili peppers and cayenne. Try some fresh lemon juice instead of vinegar on salads.

Kapha-Balancing Diet
Foods for Kapha Constitutions to Favor

General Guidelines:
- The best Kapha-balancing foods are light, dry, and warm, and have predominantly spicy, bitter, and astringent tastes. **Important secret for Kaphas:** *The bitter and astringent tastes will help curb your appetite.*
- Favor foods that are spicy and stimulating, cooked with a minimum of butter, oil, salt, and sugar.
- Always favor lightness in the diet, both in quality and quantity: smaller portions, lighter foods.

- Favor hot food over cold at every meal.
- Choose dry cooking methods (baking, broiling, sauteing) over moist or oily methods such as steaming, boiling, frying.
- Raw fruits, vegetables, and salads are recommended.

GRAINS Favor barley, buckwheat, corn, millet, rye. Basmati rice is also okay. Wheat is acceptable in small quantities.

DAIRY Only ghee (clarified butter) in small quantities and low-fat or nonfat milk are acceptable. *Hint:* To reduce the Kapha qualities of milk, you can add one or two pinches of turmeric or ginger and boil it for a few minutes. A small amount of whole milk is acceptable.

FRUITS Apples and pears are Kapha-pacifying. Apricots, cranberries, persimmons, and pomegranates are also good. Dried fruits (apricots, figs, prunes, raisins) are good for Kaphas.

VEGETABLES Almost all vegetables are Kapha-balancing, including asparagus, beets, broccoli, brussels sprouts, cabbage, carrots, cauliflower, celery, eggplant, green leafy vegetables, lettuce, peas, potatoes, pumpkin, radishes, spinach, sprouts.

NUTS Keep nuts and seeds to a minimum. Only sunflower and pumpkin seeds are acceptable in small amounts.

OILS Minimize. You can use a little almond, corn, sunflower, or safflower oil.

SWEETENERS Raw, unheated honey is the only sweetener that doesn't increase Kapha.

BEANS All are Kapha-pacifying, except tofu and kidney beans.

MEAT AND FISH Shrimp and small amounts of chicken and turkey are acceptable.

SPICES AND HERBS All spices are good for Kapha except salt. Ginger is recommended to stimulate digestion.

Eat in small quantities or avoid

General Guidelines:
- Minimize foods with heavy, oily, and cold qualities. The tastes to cut down on are sweet, sour, and salty.
- Use of dairy products should be moderate.
- Don't eat deep-fried foods.
- Avoid sweet, rich foods as much as possible.

GRAINS Only small portions of wheat and rice.

DAIRY Keep dairy products to a minimum, especially cheese, butter, and cream.

FRUITS Eat fewer sweet, very juicy, and sour fruits such as avocados, bananas, coconuts, dates, figs, grapes, melons, oranges, pineapples. These can be acceptable if cooked.

VEGETABLES Although most vegetables are good for Kapha, tomatoes, cucumbers, sweet potatoes, and zucchini are not recommended.

MEAT AND FISH Avoid pork, red meat, and seafood (except shrimp).

SPICES AND HERBS Minimize salt consumption.

Eating Out Ayurvedically

When you eat out, here are some "best and worst" foods for your constitutional type:

VATAS: Italian food, with its wheat-based pasta and creamy sauces, is excellent for Vata. Indian, Mexican, and other spicy foods are also generally good. Light-structured Vata types may want to head for the salad bar, but a heavier, warm meal would be far better. Order the soup instead of the salad, enjoy the rolls and butter, and save room for a modest-sized dessert. Lucky you—you can get away with all of that.

PITTAS: High-powered Pittas like fancy restaurants, and the pleasant environment *is* soothing to their fiery constitution. But they need to avoid Mexican and other spicy foods, and fast foods (greasy and salty) are deadly for them. Steak houses are also not the best. Try Italian (but favor the cream sauces rather than the tomatoes, and keep the cheese light), Oriental (Chinese, Japanese, Thai, etc.), or natural food restaurants. Stay away from alcohol, coffee, and hot drinks in general. Choose the salad rather than the hot soup. Desserts shouldn't be a problem.

KAPHAS: Head for the salad bar whenever you can. Otherwise, Oriental foods are generally the lightest and best for you. The spiciness of Indian food is good, and Mexican, too, if you can avoid the fried, heavier foods and cheeses. Fast foods are too oily, salty, and sweet for you. Avoid them. Ask for a cup of warm water instead of cold; watch out for the pre-meal bread and butter; choose the salad rather than the soup. Forget about the dessert if you can; if not, some fruit pie (warmed up) might be your best choice.

Ultimately, You Know Best

In addition to all the recommendations in this chapter, there is another important way to determine what you should eat and what you shouldn't. Simply put, you should eat what makes you feel good. Not just in the moment of tasting, but afterwards, too.

The "feeling good" that I'm talking about is not on the level of the senses. A lot of things feel good on the sensory level that don't pass muster deeper inside. We may do something that feels good at the moment, but deep down we know it's wrong for us. We need to listen to those inner signals. So when I say "eat what makes you feel good," I'm talking about that quieter, deeper—wiser—level of our being.

And I'm talking about the big picture, not just the moment. For instance, like Frank at the start of this chapter, you may eat something for dinner that you really enjoy, but afterwards, maybe that night or the next morning, your dullness, indigestion, or stuffed-up feeling lets you know that it wasn't such a great idea.

When people begin to become more sensitive to their bodies, perhaps through yoga, meditation, or a new attention to health, they become more aware of the effects of food on body and mind. This often leads quite spontaneously to increased use of certain foods that feel nourishing and reducing or completely dropping others that don't. Often alcohol and red meat are among the first casualties of this growing awareness.

This inner looking is an aspect of self-referral. In Chapter 1 we talked about self-referral as turning the attention to the deepest level of our being, the Self, the inner spiritual silence that is the source of our intelligence, creativity, and all that is best in us. That kind of profound self-referral is only a deeper aspect of something we do all the time, quite automatically.

You're practicing self-referral when you feel tired working out and look within to see if you should stop exercising and go home, or when you feel hungry and look inside to decide what to eat. When you're invited to get together with someone for dinner and you check with yourself to see if you want to, that inner searching around is self-referral. And when you've just *gone* to dinner and you look inside to see how you feel about the person you were with: This is self-referral too.

Most of us go into a self-referral mode for life's big decisions— "Do I really want to marry this person?" "Should I take this job?"— but we also do it for smaller issues all the time.

You can use self-referral *consciously* to learn more about what is good for you and what isn't. Simply look to see how you feel when you do certain actions or eat certain foods. For example, how do you feel when you speak sweetly to someone, as opposed to when you yell or complain? When you see a comedy or an uplifting film, as opposed to a movie full of violence and negativity? When you tell the truth as opposed to lying?

Look within, listen to yourself, pay attention to how you feel. Your inner feelings are your inner intelligence telling you what is good for you.

This habit of self-referral is one of the keys to maintaining a healthy weight. We'll talk about it in Chapter 11.

CHAPTER 4

NATURAL STRATEGIES TO DEFEAT STRESS

Stress is one of the great enemies of life. It creates tension and anxiety, robs us of happiness, comfort, creativity, love, and harmony, leads to many forms of ill health, and probably shortens our lives.

According to studies at the National Institutes of Health (NIH), approximately 90 percent of all illnesses, mental as well as physical, are caused or aggravated by stress. High blood pressure, heart disease, ulcers, and even high cholesterol are directly related to stress. It appears likely that stress destroys brain cells and weakens the immune system. Built-up stress is also at the root of psychological disorders such as insomnia, anxiety, depression, low frustration tolerance, and anger outbursts, as well as everyday tension.

Thus, this chapter on natural strategies to relieve and prevent stress is a master key to good health.

Actually, almost everything in this book can be seen as a form of stress management. Some of the suggestions, such as proper diet according to your individual constitution, balanced daily routine, and guidelines for appropriate exercise, are designed to prevent the buildup of stress by helping you toward a lifestyle more in accord with natural law.

Other approaches, such as meditation and self-massage, help to dissolve already accumulated stress. All the techniques and strategies taken as a whole can help you create a life that is free from stress and flowing in the direction of greater health and happiness.

We'll begin the chapter with a quick description of what stress is and how we acquire it. Then we'll look at proven ways to prevent and dissolve it.

Stress: The Enemy of Life

Pioneer stress researcher Dr. Hans Selye defined stress as a psycho-physiological (mind-body) event that takes place when our system is overwhelmed by any experience, whether physical, mental, or emotional. It can be long-term or sudden, something as simple as a loud noise or as complex as the continuing strain of a difficult relationship. A physical injury, or the exhaustion of trying to hold down a job and raise a family at the same time both create stress.

Stressful experiences create structural and chemical changes in the nervous system. Each accumulated stress is like a knot in the fabric of the system that impairs its normal functioning and consequently limits our mental and physical performance.

The primary cause of stress in our lives is *going against nature.*

Nature is naturally progressive, leading all her children toward growth and fulfillment. Seeds become trees, baby birds hatch and soon fly away, children grow up and take on the responsibilities of adulthood. Resisting the evolutionary flow of nature is as exhausting as swimming upstream against a strong current; going with the current, aligning our life with nature's evolutionary flow, brings health and happiness.

We get out of tune with nature in many ways—by overworking, eating the wrong foods, missing sleep, and other lifestyle choices that are not healthful and life-supporting. Our social environment contributes by providing stressful working conditions, crowded freeways, polluted air and water, and so forth.

Not respecting basic natural laws such as the need for clean air, healthful food, and adequate rest places a strain on the body that steadily builds up, weakens the system, makes us susceptible to gathering more stress, and eventually culminates in disease.

The best preventive medicine for stress is a life in accord with natural patterns and natural law. The entire program of Ayurveda is based around living life in harmony with nature, so that stress doesn't accumulate.

Suzanne, for example, regularly goes to bed by 10:30 and gets up at 6:30. She makes sure to get at least some exercise every day. Although she leads a busy life as a teacher and a mother of two, she prepares fresh natural foods whenever she can. She surrounds herself as much as possible with upbeat people and uplifting stimuli; she won't watch a violent movie and hardly ever turns on the TV. By these lifestyle choices, she is actively *creating* health.

Tom, on the other hand, has an erratic schedule that sometimes sees him going to bed in the wee hours of the morning, either because of his long hours of work or his active social life. He gets very little exercise, frequently grabs fast-food lunches, and eats a lot of packaged food at home. Tom has a strong constitution, but one look at him is enough to show that he is burning himself out by overworking and undersleeping; he is generating stress and creating the fertile ground for illness.

What can *you* do to inoculate yourself against stress?

Eight Stress-Reducing Strategies for Everyone

Here are eight powerful ways you can fight stress no matter what your body type.

1. *Follow the Ayurvedic Daily Routine.* As you will see in Chapter 6, a healthy daily routine is one of the first lines of defense against stress and one of the best things you can do for your health. Getting in tune with the rhythms of the day—waking up early in the morning as all of nature comes to life, eating your heaviest meal at midday when digestion is strongest, getting to bed early—helps you ride nature's powerful current.

Staying up late and getting overtired, eating your biggest meal at night so your digestion keeps you from sleeping well—these habits are stressful and self-defeating and eventually lead to problems. So study the chapter, reset your daily clock, and learn to go with the flow!

2. *Get Proper Exercise.* Everyone knows that a regular program of exercise is good for you. It helps keep you trim, strengthens the cardiovascular system, and is very helpful in reducing and preventing stress. What's not so well known is that improper exercise can actually *create* stress. Exercise that is the wrong kind either for your body type or for you personally, or that is too strenuous, can do more harm than good. So you've got to be careful. See Chapter 7 for details on how much and what type of exercise is most beneficial for you.

3. *Avoid Sensory Overload.* In the same way that a sudden loud noise can be stressful, a constant bombardment of loud noise is even more stressful. Any intense sensory input through any of the five senses places heavy demands on the brain and nervous system and can lead to a buildup of stress. Loud music, the rapid-fire visual input of high-action movies and TV shows, and exposure to unusual heat or cold are examples of circumstances you would be better off avoiding.

4. *Don't Get Tired.* This may sound like a joke in today's world, but you need to keep as rested as you can. Fatigue is stress on a small scale. Like stress, it prevents mind and body from functioning at their intended, normal levels. Over time, fatigue depresses the immune system, wears out the body, and produces the same harmful effects as stress.

5. *Listen to Relaxing Music.* You can use music as a kind of meditation technique. Plunk yourself down in a comfortable place, close your eyes, and listen to a tape or CD of any music that you find calming and relaxing. Classical Indian music can be very soothing. Or try the slow movement of a baroque or classical piece of music (Bach, Handel, Vivaldi, Telemann, Mozart, Haydn), or any soft and relaxing music of your choice.

6. *Take Supplements That Are Free-Radical Scavengers.* Free radicals are chemicals in our blood that can cause extensive damage to cells and tissues. They have been implicated in a wide range of conditions, including cancer, Alzheimer's disease, weakened immunity, and the degenerative processes associated with aging. Free radicals are known to be caused by pollution, improper diet—and stress.

To combat free radicals, eat foods rich in beta carotene (such as broccoli, carrots, squash, and leafy green vegetables), and take *sensible amounts* of Vitamin A, C, and E supplements. The Ayurvedic herbal formula known as *Maharishi Amrit Kalash* has also been found effective in reducing free radicals. The Japanese immunologist, Dr. Yukei Niwa, studied more than 500 substances over 30 years and found that *Amrit Kalash* was the most effective against free radicals.

7. *Play with Children.* One simple yet effective way to relieve stress is to play with children. If your life is too imbalanced in the direction of work, or if you're feeling hurried and pressured, spending some time playing with your own children, your nieces and nephews, or the children of friends can be helpful in defusing the stress. Of course, this strategy is not recommended for mothers at home, whose current stress level may have been *created* by long hours of playing with children.

8. *Make Time for Humor.* Spend some time each day doing something that makes you laugh, such as reading comics or joke books or watching hilarious videos. Taking life too seriously causes stress to build up in the system. Humor is a great way to diffuse that stress. Adding more humor to life is a common prescription made by some of the world's most renowned Ayurvedic physicians.

Stress Management for Your Body Type

In Chapter 2 you learned about body types and discovered that each of us is a unique individual with unique responses and requirements. Then you used the self-test at the end of the chapter to find out your own constitutional type. (If you haven't done so, please do that self-evaluation now; you really won't be able to use most of the strategies suggested in this book unless you know your body type.)

In Chapter 3 you built on this knowledge, learning how to develop an appropriate, personalized eating plan. Now let's see how the three main body types respond to stressful circumstances and how each can guard against stress.

Strategies to Prevent and Relieve Stress for Vata Types

People with Vata constitutions are particularly prone to Vata stress, but anyone can fall prey to Vata symptoms. Long exposure to cold or windy weather, lack of regular daily habits, fatigue, prolonged worry or anxiety, fasting, or an extremely light diet are among the many conditions that encourage excess Vata to build up.

Some of the ways Vata-related stress manifests itself include insomnia, anxiety or fear, acting "hyper," overtalkativeness, heart palpitations, constipation alternating with diarrhea (a common condition known as "irritable bowel syndrome"), nervous stomach, feeling cold easily (especially in the hands and feet), feeling faint or dizzy, and high blood pressure. If you have any of these symptoms, the following strategies will be helpful to you.

- A good daily routine is extremely important for settling aggravated Vata. This is especially true of an *early bedtime*—something that may be quite difficult for the impulsive Vata personality to achieve, but which is very balancing and valuable.

- Sip warm or hot water often during the day (warm in hot weather, otherwise hot).

- Drink a cup of warm milk brewed with a teaspoon of poppy seeds, especially at bedtime. Instead of poppy seeds, you can use a pinch of cardamom or a *small* pinch of nutmeg.

- Give yourself a massage with sesame oil. (See the instructions for performing the self-massage—known in Ayurveda as *abhyanga*—in the box on pages 58–60.) If insomnia is troubling you, you can get some of the same benefits by rubbing a little sesame oil or ghee on your feet before you go to bed. Massage each foot for about five minutes. Rub the entire foot, but concentrate especially on the soles. Finish by wiping with a cool cloth.

- Take the herb *gotu kola,* either in capsules or as a tea. Take up to half a teaspoon steeped in a cup of hot water, with a little honey added after your tea cools enough to drink. Gotu kola is available in most natural food stores.

- A ready-made tea, blended of Vata-pacifying herbs and also available in most natural foods stores, is Maharishi Ayur-Veda's "Vata Tea." (See Appendix C for a list of herb sources.)

- Take a warm bath or shower.

- Get some mild exercise, such as walking, yoga, or easy bicycle riding. Strenuous exercise can aggravate Vata, especially in a person with a predominantly Vata body type.

SOOTHE AWAY STRESSES
WITH AYURVEDIC SELF-MASSAGE

Ayurvedic self-massage, using warm oil, is a great way to relax and dissolve stress and tension. Rubbing the oil into your head, body, and feet is as soothing as it is enjoyable. But it also accomplishes something more, building a kind of "psychological immunity" to stress by giving you a flexible, relaxed frame of mind and body to help you deal with life's difficult moments. The more relaxed you are when you face a potentially stressful situation, the better you'll be able to deal with it, without creating more stress for yourself.

Ideally, you'll do the *abhyanga* or oil massage first thing in the morning as part of the Ayurvedic morning routine recommended in Chapter 6. You can also give yourself a massage at night, if you are having trouble relaxing and getting to sleep.

Here's what to do:

First you'll have to buy the oil. For most people, refined sesame oil is best, cold pressed and pure, not the flavored Chinese kind used for cooking. If it irritates your skin (a possibility if you are a Pitta, as sesame has warming properties), you may use olive oil or coconut oil.

Next, set up the spot where you'll do your massages. The best place is the bathroom, because no matter how careful you are, you'll probably get some oil on the floor. I recommend using a sheet of plastic (perhaps a large trash bag) directly on the bathroom floor; then place a towel on top of that to sit on more comfortably. Keep the towel for just this purpose, and whenever you wash it, be careful to dry it on low temperature in an automatic dryer, or better, hang it up to dry either indoors or out. The reason: the oil can be a fire hazard.

Next, warm up the oil. Use only about a quarter cup—about three or four tablespoons. Heat for just a few seconds on the stove, or place it in a cup or plastic squeeze bottle in some warm water. Place a few drops on the back of your hand to make sure it's not too hot.

Then begin the massage. Start with your head. Rub about a tablespoonful into your scalp, using your palms, *not* your fingertips. Use small circular strokes to rub in the oil, and you can rub quite vigorously here.

Next do your forehead, face, and neck. Here the pressure should be more gentle. Use a back-and-forth motion on your forehead. Pay particular attention to the temples (very soothing to Vata), using a circular motion, and to the outside of the ears.

Reach behind and massage the upper part of the back and spine, and the backs of your shoulders.

Proceed to your shoulders and arms, where you'll use a long motion, straight back and forth over the long bones, and a circular motion over the joints. Here again, vigorous strokes are appropriate.

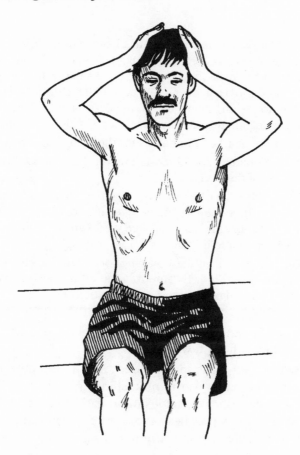

Lighten up again as you massage your chest and trunk. Use a straight up-and-down motion over the center of the chest (sternum), and a circular motion on the breasts and again over the stomach and lower abdomen.

Reach around and massage your lower back as well as you can.

Vigorous strokes are good for the legs, again using a circular motion on the joints (knees and ankles) and a straight back-and-forth motion on the long bones.

Finally, massage your feet. Like Chinese medicine and Reflexology, Ayurveda considers the feet very important, so take some time. Use the flat of your hand to rub the soles of your feet rather vigorously and then use your fingers to work around the toes.

When you've finished the massage, leave the oil on your skin as long as you can, but be sure to rub off the excess before you bathe, to prevent clogging the drain.

(Box text continues on page 60)

Tips:

1. For best results, use oil that has been "cured," that is, heated to 212° F. You can cure up to a quart at a time, which will be enough for about 15 massages. Place the oil in a pan with a drop or two of water on top. Heat over a low heat until the drop of water boils or turns to steam, then quickly remove oil from heat. Important: When heating the oil, stay by the stove. Oils are flammable.

2. Allow about 10 to 15 minutes for the complete massage.

3. Proportionately, spend more time on the head and feet than on the rest of the body.

4. If you don't have time for the complete massage, you can do a two- or three-minute "mini" massage, emphasizing your head and feet. For this mini massage, you can sit on the edge of the tub for a couple of minutes before bathing.

5. *Safety note:* Oil on the bottom of your feet increases the risk of slipping in the tub. Be sure to wipe off as much as you can before getting into the water and be extra careful.

- Dip a washcloth in warm water and place it over your forehead and eyes for a few minutes.

- Follow the Vata-pacifying diet described in Chapter 3. Concentrate on food that is warm, nourishing, and easy to digest. Add some ghee to your vegetables or spread it on bread. Eat sweet, juicy fruit such as peaches. Avoid dry fruit or apples, which increase Vata. Have some warm milk as a snack.

- The scents of frankincense, basil, orange, and clove are soothing to Vata. These fragrances can be diffused into the air as incense or in the form of an aroma oil.

Strategies to Prevent and Relieve Stress for Pitta Types

Typical symptoms of Pitta-related stress are anger or irritability, feeling heat in the body, skin rashes, eye irritation, burning in the rectal area, acid stomach or heartburn, and an intolerance to heat. Here are some simple, natural ways to combat Pitta stress and keep the volatile Pitta nature from exploding:

- Follow the Pitta-pacifying diet, favoring sweet foods or foods that are bitter or astringent, such as a salad with leafy green vegetables. In a situation of acute stress, drink a glass of cold water or have some ice cream. It may sound simplistic, but it works.

- Place a washcloth dipped in cold water over your forehead and eyes for a few minutes.
- Rose-petal jam, made with brown sugar, is very soothing to Pitta, as are a few drops of rose water in a glass of water and lightly sweetened. Maharishi Ayur-Veda has a delicious rose-petal jam available at many natural food stores.
- Make some tea using the herbs fennel and coriander. Add one quarter teaspoon of each herb to two glasses of water. Boil down to one half the amount of water. Strain out the herbs, then add unrefined sugar or another natural sweetener and let cool. (If you use honey, don't add it until the tea is cool enough to drink.) You can add a little milk or cream.
- A ready-made tea blended of Pitta-pacifying herbs, available in most natural foods stores, is Maharishi Ayur-Veda's "Pitta Tea."
- Still another good drink is licorice tea. Please note: All teas for Pitta body types should be taken warm in cool weather or at room temperature to slightly cool in warm weather.
- Ghee is the most Pitta-pacifying food substance. Spread some on toast or add a spoonful to a cup of room-temperature milk.
- Take a cool bath or shower.
- Go swimming or skiing. Don't do exercises that heat you up a lot or that stimulate intense competitive feelings.
- Give yourself an oil massage, but instead of sesame oil, which is warming, use coconut oil.
- Use some sterile saline solution, available in any drugstore, as eye drops. Place a couple of drops of the cool (not cold) liquid in each eye.
- A simple breathing exercise to cool the system is to breathe through the left nostril only. Place your right thumb over your right nostril and breath normally through the left nostril for five to ten minutes. Don't force it if the nostril is clogged.
- Sandalwood, rose, lavender, and jasmine scents are cooling to Pitta. These can be diffused into the air as incense or aroma oil.

Strategies to Prevent and Relieve Stress for Kapha Types

The naturally more serene, "laid-back" character of Kaphas makes them more resistant to stressful situations than the hyperactive Vata or the irascible Pitta. But Kapha types also incur stress under difficult circumstances. When they do, they tend to accumulate more Kapha.

Kapha generally increases due to a combination of eating too much, consuming too many oily and/or sweet foods, and lack of exercise.

In such situations, a person whose constitution is already weighted toward Kapha tends to lose ambition and motivation. This is where the couch-potato syndrome can make its appearance. Depression is common, as are feelings or behaviors expressing greediness and possessiveness.

- The best antidote for Kapha stress is to eat light, dry foods, emphasizing fruits, vegetables, lentils, and light grains such as rye and barley.
- A vegetarian diet is ideal, but lean turkey or chicken are all right if you feel the need for meat.
- Tofu or warm skim milk (with a little ginger and turmeric added) are good protein supplements to a vegetarian diet.
- One day each week, eat very lightly, taking just soups, teas, skim milk, fruit, and juices throughout the day, avoiding solid food.
- Regular exercise, gradually increasing the amount over time, will be helpful in combatting Kapha stress.

Nearly all the recommendations in the preceding pages are free or cost only a few dollars for some herbs or oils. These suggestions are as useful for prevention as they are for cure. Take advantage of these natural remedies and preventive measures to keep your life in balance.

Two Natural Relaxation Techniques

Before we explore several powerful Ayurvedic methods of stress reduction, I'd like to introduce you to a couple of modern Western methods that are being used with great success. Both are entirely natural and can be learned in more detail from a book or audio tape, though the following points may provide enough information for you to try them now.

Dissolve Muscle Tension Fast.

"Progressive Relaxation" is a technique in which you systematically tighten and then relax various muscle groups while breathing deeply from the diaphragm. Some of the audio tapes that teach it have some soothing background music accompanying the instructions.

Basically, this is what you do: Sit comfortably or lie on your back on your bed or on a mat or blanket on the floor. Begin by closing your eyes and focusing for a few minutes on your breathing. Breathe slowly and deeply from your belly or diaphragm. You can test this by placing your hand on your abdomen, with the little finger over the navel. When you're breathing correctly, you'll feel your hand rising and falling.

The next phase involves tensing and relaxing your muscles from your feet to your head. As you move from area to area, place your full attention there; tense all the muscles; inhale and hold for several seconds, then exhale as you let go of the tension; enjoy the relaxation for several seconds before moving on.

Begin by tensing the muscles in your left foot, ankle, and toes for a few seconds, then relax them. Tighten your left calf muscles for a few seconds, and relax. Then repeat these steps with your right foot and leg.

Gradually proceed upward, flexing and releasing muscles and muscle groups, from your legs and thighs to the muscles of the buttocks, abdomen, chest, back, shoulders, arms (one at a time, as with your legs and feet) and, finally, the muscles of your neck, jaws, and face. Then just lie quietly for a few minutes and enjoy the relaxed feeling.

Take an Instant Vacation with Guided Imagery.

A session of guided imagery usually begins with deep breathing, listening to music, or with some other way to promote a relaxed state. Once some degree of relaxation is achieved, begin to imagine a scene that has pleasant associations for you, such as a secluded meadow in the mountains with a stream running through it; lying on the beach feeling the warm sunshine; or sitting by the shore at sunset. Using all your senses—imagining how it feels, smells, sounds, and so on—increases the effectiveness of the exercise and deepens the level of relaxation.

Use Guided Imagery to Relieve Pain.

A variation of the technique I just described can also be helpful for controlling pain. Some patients in progressive pain clinics around the country are learning to mentally direct healing imagery to the area of their discomfort. Mike, a metal worker who had injured his back in a fall, used the technique to visualize a golden energy flowing over the irritated nerves in his back. After he practiced awhile and mastered the process, he felt a great deal of relief.

Guided imagery appears to have been instrumental even in the healing of several cancer patients, as indicated by the famous—and controversial—research of O. Carl Simonton, M.D. For best results, consult with a therapist professionally trained in self-hypnosis and guided imagery. He or she will be able to teach you a step-by-step process and provide guidance to ensure greater success in the practice.

Breathe Away Tensions

For thousands of years, the Vedic breathing exercises known as *pranayama* have been used to reduce stress and calm the system. The secret of their effectiveness is that breathing provides an instant hookup with the brain. The center that regulates breathing, in the part of the brain known as the medulla, also governs the other automatic functions of the physiology, such as heart rate. It is intimately related to the autonomic nervous system, which directs bodily functions such as digestion and metabolism.

Breathing has always been considered very important in Ayurveda because it brings *prana* (life energy) into our system from the environment. Prana is vital to life; it is vitality itself. The following rhythmical breathing exercise helps to bring that life energy into the body in a more efficient way, producing a sense of vitality and energy. It also increases the amount of oxygen in the blood. Proper oxygenation is critical to life because every cell in the body depends on a sufficient oxygen supply in order to function properly.

Alternate-nostril breathing, as in the following exercise, balances all three doshas and helps organize the brain to become more coherent. By making the respiratory rhythm more regular, it helps to generate a soothing influence for the entire nervous system.

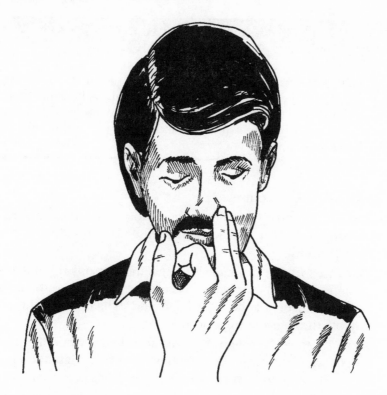

The Balancing Breath. Perform this easy breathing exercise while you are sitting down. Balanced breathing is relaxing, helps to integrate mind and body, and creates a state of peacefulness and inner calm. If you use it for about five minutes before your morning and afternoon meditation sessions, you will find that you settle into meditation more quickly and deeply.

Balanced breathing is not deep breathing. Just breathe normally and naturally. You might even find that your breath becomes shallower as you relax. This is fine.

You will be using the thumb, middle, and ring fingers of your right hand for this exercise.

Step One: Sit comfortably with your back in an upright position. It is better not to be leaning back. Keep your neck and head free.

HOW TO REDUCE ANGER AND ANXIETY BY BREATHING

According to Ayurveda, breathing through the left nostril has a cooling effect. It is good for reducing Pitta, irritability, and anger. Breathing through the right nostril has a warming effect, which helps pacify Vata, reduces anxiety, and creates calmness. It also reduces Kapha by gently stimulating *agni,* the digestive fire.

Step Two: Close your eyes.

Step Three: Inhale normally, then close your right nostril by pressing against it with your right thumb and exhale through the left nostril.

Step Four: Inhale normally through the left nostril, and when the inhalation is complete, close the left nostril with the middle and ring fingers of the right hand and exhale easily and comfortably through the right nostril.

Step Five: Inhale through the right nostril, and when the inhalation is complete, close the right nostril with the right thumb and exhale through the left nostril. This completes one cycle.

Step Six: Continue repeating this cycle for five minutes, switching nostrils after each inhalation and keeping your breathing comfortable, continuous, and steady.

The Ultimate Stress-Management Technique

The most powerful stress-management tool I know of is meditation. An effective meditation technique releases built-up tension and relaxes both mind and body simultaneously. This makes us feel better immediately and allows us to relate to the world in a more easygoing yet clear-minded manner.

Several meditation techniques have been found useful in promoting relaxation, reducing anxiety, and creating a greater sense of well-being. One such technique, popularized by a number of teachers including Jon Kabat-Zinn, M.D., at the University of Massachusetts, is called "Mindfulness Meditation." Dr. Kabat-Zinn's books, *Full Catastrophe Living* and his later volume, *Wherever I Go, There I*

Am, explain the practice and contain moving descriptions of some of its results.

Although there are a number of techniques of meditation being taught today, Transcendental Meditation is by far the most thoroughly researched in terms of its benefits for mental, physical, and social health. It also has the endorsement of the American Association of Ayurvedic Medicine. TM is a simple mental technique, easy to learn and practice. Anyone can learn it within a few days and can begin to experience beneficial results almost immediately.

Tim is a 48-year-old senior vice president of a large insurance company. Although highly successful in his career, he had never learned how to relax, which affected the quality of his work relationships and his personal life as well. He found himself relying more and more on alcohol and cigarettes to calm his nerves and "wind down" at the end of a hard day. His mood was generally tense and with increasing frequency he found himself getting irritated without much cause. He became especially worried when his wife started complaining that he wasn't the same person she married 20 years earlier. She was beginning to talk about divorce.

A co-worker and longtime friend of Tim's happened to have learned TM a few months previously and was finding it to be a useful stress-reduction tool in her own life. She recommended TM and suggested that Tim go to a free introductory talk at the local library to learn more about it. Although he was openly skeptical, Tim ended up taking the TM course; to his pleasant surprise, his life began to turn around.

In his own words, "I couldn't believe how simple it was. The very first day I learned, I felt as if a weight was lifted off my shoulders. Colors seemed brighter, I noticed the birds singing—it was great! And each day I seem to discover a new benefit. Some days it's something simple, like not getting irritated in a traffic jam. I find that I organize my work more efficiently, and I'm a lot more patient in dealing with people at the office. Dropping so much stress has also given me more energy.

"I usually stay later than most people at the office. Since learning TM, I generally shut my door and spend my last 20 minutes there meditating, before going home. One evening I realized that I had gone home, sat down, and started talking to my wife; a couple of hours had passed and I hadn't poured myself a drink. I just forgot! I felt so relaxed I didn't feel the need for it, and since then I've become an occasional social drinker instead of a man who always—and I mean always—had a few drinks in the afternoon and evening. The change is just terrific."

TM was brought to the Western world in the 1950s by Maharishi Mahesh Yogi and is now taught throughout the world by thousands of teachers trained by this Indian sage. It is practiced for a few minutes twice a day with eyes closed while sitting in a comfortable position, whether on a chair, on the couch, or wherever you're most relaxed. During the practice the mind settles to its most quiet level, and the body simultaneously receives a deep state of rest.

More than a decade ago, stress expert Hans Selye said,

> Research already conducted shows that the physiological effects of Transcendental Meditation are exactly the opposite to those identified by medicine as being characteristic of the body's effort to meet the demands of stress. The TM technique is a method which so relaxes the human central nervous system that . . . it doesn't suffer from stress.

Over 500 scientific studies have been performed on TM at major American universities and research institutes from Harvard to UCLA, and in more than 35 countries. The earliest research, published in 1970, showed that the entire physical system received a very deep rest. Heart rate slowed, breathing became slower, blood pressure lowered, and the metabolic rate dropped 15 percent or more within a few minutes after starting meditation, as compared with a drop of about 10 percent during deep sleep.

This is very important, because rest is such a vital factor in healing. For centuries, physicians have advised their patients to rest when they are sick. Rest allows the body to throw off stress and most efficiently heal itself. When the body is resting, all its energy and intelligence can be applied toward the healing process rather than expended for other activities and processes.

It makes sense that deeper rest permits more self-repair and rejuvenation. The state of *absolute rest* created by the mental stillness of meditation enlivens the body's inner intelligence and enables our self-healing, stress-dissolving mechanisms to become most effective.

Later studies on TM showed that the restful levels of functioning produced by the practice persist and stabilize *outside* the meditation period as a person meditates regularly for several years. This means that the whole system begins to operate at a more efficient level, outwardly dynamic while remaining inwardly restful. This produces a growing sense of inner calm and balance, a spiritual centeredness that builds a kind of "psychological immunity" to stress.

"The best thing about meditation for me," said Jeanine, a 42-year-old secretary and mother of three who has been meditating for about six years, "is the inner evenness I feel. No matter what comes up, at home or at work, I seem to be able to deal with it without getting thrown this way or that. I'm basically a pretty emotional person, and this is a big change for me. I used to get more upset than most people. Even little things used to bother me a lot. Now, even though my life is about as hectic as ever, I just kind of flow along."

Research has shown that hormones and other biochemical compounds in the blood indicative of stress tend to decrease during TM practice. These changes also stabilize over time, so that a person is actually less stressed *biochemically* during daily activity.

This reduction of stress translates directly into a reduction of anxiety and tension. Literally dozens of studies have shown this. One researcher, Kenneth Eppley of Stanford University, performed a "meta-analysis," comparing 99 different studies on the effects of various kinds of meditation and relaxation techniques on anxiety. A number of the techniques did significantly reduce anxiety. However, Eppley found that TM was about twice as effective as the other forms.

More and more physicians are recommending TM because, in addition to the vast amount of research on it, it is taught in a systematic and reliable way by teachers who have been thoroughly trained.

TM is one of the few recommendations in this book that cannot be taught to you in these pages. In order to gain maximum benefit from the practice, personal instruction from a qualified teacher is necessary. Virtually all major cities on all five continents have TM centers where you can take the four-day course that will enable you to become proficient and self-sufficient in this practice.

One word of advice: After you learn TM, periodically get your meditation practice "checked" by your TM instructor. These periodic

18 BENEFITS OF TRANSCENDENTAL MEDITATION

Here is a summary of some of the main benefits of TM for mind and body as discovered by research in the past 25 years:

Physical Benefits

- Deep rest—as measured by decreased metabolic rate, lower heart rate, and reduced work load of the heart.
- Lowered levels of cortisol and lactate—two chemicals associated with stress.
- Reduction of free radicals—unstable oxygen molecules that can cause tissue damage. They are now thought to be a major factor in aging and in many diseases.
- Decreased high blood pressure.
- Higher skin resistance. Low skin resistance is correlated with higher stress and anxiety levels.
- Drop in cholesterol levels. High cholesterol is associated with cardio-vascular disease.
- Improved flow of air to the lungs resulting in easier breathing. This has been very helpful to asthma patients.
- Younger biological age. On standard measures of aging, long-term TM practitioners (more than five years) measured 12 years younger than their chronological age.
- Higher levels of DHEAS in the elderly. An additional sign of youthful-ness through TM; lower levels of DHEAS are associated with aging.

Psychological Benefits

- Increased brain wave coherence. Harmony of brain wave activity in different parts of the brain is associated with greater creativity, im-proved moral reasoning, and higher IQ.
- Decreased anxiety.
- Decreased depression.
- Decreased irritability and moodiness.
- Improved learning ability and memory.
- Increased self-actualization.
- Increased feelings of vitality and rejuvenation.
- Increased happiness.
- Increased emotional stability.

tune-ups keep the practice effortless and most effective, resulting in the most benefits.

Dealing with Extreme Stress

In addition to the "routine" stresses of daily life, some people experience very upsetting events that can result in what is now called post-traumatic stress disorder (PTSD). War, rape or other sexual abuse, serious accidents, or exposure to natural disasters such as earthquakes can have a lasting negative effect on a person's life.

Dealing with the aftermath of these extraordinarily stressful circumstances calls for some help from a mental health professional. But in addition, the stress-management techniques suggested in this chapter will help to soothe and dissolve such high levels of stress. In particular, the TM technique is recommended.

Tom Scarano, Ph.D., and James S. Brooks, M.D. (co-author of this book) studied the effects of TM on Vietnam veterans who were suffering from a high degree of stress. We found a significant reduction in depression, anxiety, alcohol consumption, and other PTSD symptoms. I believe that if TM can help reduce the devastating load of stress these ex-soldiers were carrying around, it can certainly help the rest of us deal with the less dramatic stress of our daily lives.

Potentially stressful situations are surely unavoidable in life, but how we deal with them is largely up to us. If you make use of the suggestions and techniques in this chapter you will have a personal stress-management system strong enough to help you deal gracefully with whatever life sends your way.

CHAPTER 5

HOW TO STRENGTHEN YOUR IMMUNE SYSTEM AND STAY HEALTHY

Why is it that out of 100 people exposed to a cold or flu virus, only a few may actually "catch" it? We all breathe in millions of germs every day, yet nobody falls prey to *all* these germs, and some people almost never get sick. What's the difference between those who get sick often and those who seem to be almost invincible?

The answer lies primarily in the immune system. If your immunity is strong you will rarely get sick. Ayurvedic medicine, which is highly prevention-oriented, recommends numerous strategies to help you keep your immunity strong so you can prevent illnesses of all kinds. In this chapter we'll look at several of these powerful recommendations.

Ojas: Your Body's Secret Key to Immunity

In Ayurvedic medicine a person's immunity is based primarily on the strength of his or her *ojas*. To understand what ojas is, we need to look at an important aspect of Ayurvedic physiology we have not yet considered: the *dhatus*.

Ayurveda holds that the human body is constructed of seven basic tissues:

1. Plasma (*rasa*) contains the nutritive product of digestion and nourishes all bodily tissues and organs.
2. Red blood cells (*rakta*) govern the body's ability to use oxygen.
3. Muscle (*mamsa*) maintains physical strength.
4. Fat (*meda*) lubricates the system.
5. Bone (*asthi*) supports the body structure.
6. Bone marrow and nerves (*majja*) form the material of brain and nervous system.
7. Reproductive tissue (*shukra*) is responsible for reproduction and the production of ojas.

The dhatus or bodily tissues are formed sequentially, each dependent on the one previous to it. The shukra or reproductive tissue (which includes all the reproductive fluids and hormones, testosterone, semen, ovum, and so forth) is thus the end product or high point of a long process of development. As such it is considered to be made up of a very refined material, vitally important for optimum functioning of the brain, the nervous system, and the immune system.

Ojas, which is said to be derived from shukra, confers mental, spiritual, and physical strength. A person with abundant ojas has a sharp, clear mind, a strong and flexible body, and spiritual power. He or she is naturally attractive and charismatic, due to an almost palpable radiance or glow. Someone with plentiful ojas is vital and vibrant and spontaneously expresses love, warmth, calmness, and creativity.

Ojas nourishes the body's organs as well as the finer emotions. It promotes vitality and a high level of mental, emotional, and physical health. Some Ayurvedic authorities say that ojas is the essence of life and that when ojas is completely depleted, the person dies.

When ojas does become weak or reduced, vitality is lowered and all the qualities associated with lack of life energy begin to make their appearance. Creativity and joy of life are dampened, and depression may set in.

Perhaps most important from a health standpoint, weakened ojas allows the digestive fire (*agni*) to become diminished. With weakened agni, digestion becomes less effective, leaving the undigested and partially digested materials that Ayurveda refers to as *ama,* or impurities. As we will discuss in greater detail in Chapter 10, ama is the fertile breeding ground for all sorts of diseases.

Thus we need to keep ojas abundant. The following factors reduce ojas and should be avoided as much as possible:

- Anything that aggravates or increases Vata, such as irregular schedule, Vata-increasing foods, etc.
- Travel, especially over several time zones. If you do travel a lot, take care to get extra rest to help your body compensate for the strain of jet lag.
- Stale, old, processed, or other forms of junk food with little life in it.
- Too much exercise for your body type.
- Too much sex, including masturbation.
- Fasting too long or too often.
- Negative emotions such as fear, worry, envy, anger, grief, etc.
- Overwork.
- Constant hurrying.
- Illness or injury.

Some factors that increase ojas include:

- Balanced lifestyle according to your body type.
- Meditation.
- Foods such as milk, ghee, rice, honey.
- Rejuvenative herbs such as the Indian herbs *ashvagandha* (winter cherry) and *shatavari* (Indian asparagus).
- Sexual moderation or abstinence.

Producing and maintaining abundant ojas is the most important way to a strong immune system.

Build Immunity on the Three Pillars of Life

According to Ayurveda, the three pillars of life and good health are proper nutrition, adequate rest, and conservation of sexual energy. If these three are properly taken care of, immunity will naturally be strong, health will be vibrant, and life will be long.

The first pillar: Nutrition

Nourish yourself with fresh, pure food that creates balance in your system. Follow the diet plan for your constitutional type suggested in Chapter 3, but for best results be sure to take into consideration the season of the year as well as your body type.

Also, to create balance and avoid food cravings, be sure to include all six tastes in every meal. (The six tastes, described in Chapter 3, are sweet, sour, salty, bitter, astringent, and pungent or spicy.) Follow the guidelines in Chapter 10 for maximizing digestion, such as eating lightly at night, taking your largest meal at lunchtime, eating moderate portions, and so on.

Stay away from stale, heavy food that is difficult to digest and that generates ama. Try to keep away from food that would produce an imbalance in your system. For example, minimize Vata-increasing foods such as salads and cold or drying foods if you are a Vata type, refrain from Pitta-increasing foods in hot weather, and so on.

The second pillar: Adequate rest

You've probably experienced many times that you're most susceptible to getting sick when you let yourself get tired. Getting enough rest is essential not only to good health and strong immunity, but to a clear mind and positive feelings. It's hard to deal with difficult situations and turn a cheerful face to difficult people when you're feeling worn down.

Ayurveda not only suggests getting enough rest, it also tells you *when* to get it, *how much* you need, and provides many suggestions to help you get good, deep sleep. (See Chapter 12.)

As you will see in the next chapter, every day nature goes through two cycles of Vata, Pitta, and Kapha influence:

First Cycle	*Second Cycle*
6 A.M. to 10 A.M. = Kapha	6 P.M. to 10 P.M. = Kapha
10 A.M. to 2 P.M. = Pitta	10 P.M. to 2 A.M. = Pitta
2 P.M. to 6 P.M. = Vata	2 A.M. to 6 A.M. = Vata

If you go to bed during the Kapha phase of the cycle in the evening, ideally between 9 P.M. and 10 P.M. when the heavy Kapha influence is increasing and then dominating, you will fall asleep more easily, sleep more deeply, and feel rested in the morning. And if you wake up before the morning Kapha phase begins (before 6 A.M.) you will carry the lightness and clarity of the Vata influence with you all day.

Remember also that the different body types need different amounts of sleep. If you are predominantly a Kapha, you may require up to eight or nine hours of sleep in order to feel rested. Pittas need seven or eight, and Vatas generally feel fine with six or seven.

This is only a rough guideline, however. Each of us is unique, and our sleep needs will vary. They will also vary at different stages of our lives. As we get older, for instance, all body types tend more toward Vata. At that time our sleep needs may decrease and our sleep patterns change toward the light, interrupted Vata style of sleeping.

Getting enough rest also means not burning yourself out with overactivity. That could mean overextending yourself at work, over-exerting in exercise, or trying to do too much, not pacing yourself, or burning the candle at both ends. Be careful. Exhaustion is one of the quickest ways to reduce ojas and weaken your immunity.

The third pillar: Conservation of sexual energy

The third way to increase ojas and build immunity is by conservation of sexual energy. As we will see later in the book (Chapter 18), Ayurveda has a unique and helpful understanding of sex. One aspect of this understanding is that the different body types have different sexual "capacities" and inclinations, which need to be respected to maintain good health.

Kaphas, while slower to be aroused, can enjoy much more sexual activity before becoming tired or satiated; Pittas, while usually passionate, have an intermediate level of sexual energy; and Vatas, quickly excited and quickly satiated, can tolerate the least sexual activity and easily become drained and exhausted by too much sex.

As we saw at the beginning of the chapter, ojas, the central player in the strength of the immune system, depends on shukra, the sexual fluids, for nourishment. When shukra is depleted due to too much sexual activity, ojas becomes weak and the immune system is compromised. Many people have experienced that they tend to be more susceptible to colds or the flu when they overindulge in sex; this is the reason why.

The Ayurvedic recommendation regarding sex, if you want to sustain maximum immunity, is moderation. If you are sick, total abstinence for a few weeks or even longer will help you build up strength. But in general, moderation according to your body type is best. That means Kaphas can indulge most, Vatas least. And, contrary to Western medical theory, being inclined toward celibacy is considered a positive and healthy lifestyle choice.

Five More Ways You Can Build Your Immunity

Ayurveda offers many more suggestions to maintain strong immunity. Here are five additional strategies to help you stay healthy.

Get enough exercise

The value of exercise for enhancing immunity has become quite well known and accepted in Western medicine in the past several decades. Researchers have found that endorphins (the body's natural painkillers) increase during exercise and that there is a definite correlation between increased endorphins and increased immunity.

From an Ayurvedic point of view, exercise

- improves digestion and assimilation,
- clears toxins out of the system,
- reduces stress and helps to dissolve negative feelings,
- promotes sound sleep,
- increases energy and stamina,

all of which strengthen our immunity.

Once again it is important to emphasize that you need to determine the type, amount, and intensity of exercise you do with reference to your body type. Kaphas need a good aerobic workout several times a week. Pittas need moderate levels of exercise but should avoid intense competition and overheating, both of which aggravate Pitta. Vatas usually need only mild exercise such as walking, yoga postures, or dancing, so long as it's not too strenuous.

Not getting enough exercise allows ama to accumulate in the body, which reduces immunity. On the other hand, overexerting in exercise produces fatigue, which also compromises the immune system. So find the right balance for you and stick with it.

Keep your emotions as positive as possible

As Deepak Chopra, M.D., has pointed out, we actually *make* the body with our thoughts and feelings. The contemporary science known as psycho-neuro-immunology (the science of how the mind or psyche influences the immune system) has demonstrated that our thoughts produce molecules that then structure our bodies.

When we think positive, optimistic, happy thoughts, we produce "happy" molecules—specific molecules that are different from the chemicals produced by unhappy, angry, or depressed thoughts and feelings. What we think, we become—literally. This is very important because happiness produces a biochemistry that strengthens immunity, while unhappiness and depression suppress our immune system's effectiveness.

So, as much as you can, put your attention on the positive and be as happy as you can be. Playing with children, reading uplifting books, encouraging laughter by reading comics or watching comedies, and so on, are all helpful activities to promote immunity.

Sip hot water

One of the body's great invitations to disease is ama. The more ama we have accumulated in our system, the more likely we are to get sick. One simple, natural way to reduce ama and clear it out of the body, suggested by Maharishi Ayur-Veda physicians, is to drink a few sips of hot water frequently throughout the day. You can do this routinely (except in very hot weather or if you are very Pitta in your constitution), and especially if you are prone to colds or feel a cold coming on. Take a few sips of hot water about once every half hour.

Neutralize stress through meditation

It is now well known medically that stress weakens immune functioning, but most of us have already learned this from our own experience. When we're exhausted or under a lot of work pressure or emotional strain, we seem to get sick much more readily. Mental techniques that reduce stress can therefore be very helpful to increase immune functioning and prevent illnesses from arising.

Spend some time every day practicing Transcendental Meditation, which is most thoroughly researched in terms of proven effectiveness, or any other effective technique you may have learned. TM research has demonstrated that regularly reducing stress results in prevention of illness through the enhancement of immune functioning. Refer to Chapter 4 for further suggestions.

Use strengthening and cleansing herbs

Both rejuvenating herbs and cleansing herbs can play a vital role in enhancing immunity. Rejuvenating herbs such as *ashvagandha* (winter cherry) and *shatavari* (Indian asparagus) nourish the system. *Gotu kola* has been called "perhaps the most important rejuvenative herb in Ayurvedic medicine" by Dr. Vasant Lad and Dr. David Frawley in their outstanding reference book, *The Yoga of Herbs*. This herb is not only good for the nerves and brain cells, but is a blood purifier that both cleanses and fortifies the immune system.

An herbal mixture combining all three of these rejuvenating herbs is Maharishi Ayur-Veda's "Almond Energy." (Almonds are also considered to be very strengthening for the brain and nervous system.) These tonifying herbs counteract any weakness in the body.

Cleansing herbs can also play a key role in improving your immunity. Because so much illness results from inadequate digestion and the subsequent accumulation of ama in the body, purifying the system to remove the ama has a direct effect on increasing immunity. In this regard some of the heating herbs are very powerful, including ginger, black pepper, and the Indian herb known as *pippali* or Indian long pepper. These three mixed in equal proportions form an inexpensive and effective compound known as *trikatu,* which is excellent for cleansing the system of ama as well as stimulating the digestive fires.

Other useful herbs include basil, bayberry, and wild yam root (which contains *dioscorea villosa,* a precursor to the anti-aging substance DHEA). Garlic is a rejuvenative that also cleanses the blood, but is very heating and can act as an irritant so should be used with some caution.

Several herbal compounds can also be useful for strengthening immunity, primarily the Ayurvedic compound called *chyavanprash,* the main ingredient of which is *amalak* fruit, famous for its high Vitamin C content. An herbal mixture similar to *chyavanprash,* known as *Maharishi Amrit Kalash*, has been subjected to laboratory tests and found effective in combating cancer cells, reducing cholesterol, and increasing endorphins in laboratory conditions. Another excellent and inexpensive compound is *triphala,* which has both cleansing and tonic properties.

Your body's immune system is a crucial factor in keeping you healthy and disease free. Use the many tips in this chapter to enhance your immunity and gain increasing vitality and freedom from disease.

CHAPTER 6

LIVING IN TUNE WITH NATURE
DAILY AND SEASONAL ROUTINES

The Rhythms of Life

Each day the earth transforms itself gracefully, moving from pre-dawn darkness to first light, then the golden rising sun, high noon, sunset, dusk, and a return to darkness. The year, too, flows from season to season, undergoing massive changes. Cold winter, with its short days and long, dark nights, its icy winds and subdued color scheme, gives way to the riot of energy that is spring. Summer is not far behind, heating the earth and bringing crops to fruition. And then comes autumn, with its blazing colors, crisp air, and falling leaves as the year settles toward winter and another cycle of rest.

Year after year, century after century, age after age, all of nature repeats this timeless rhythm. And within these great cycles are countless lesser ones. Animals go to sleep at dusk and awaken at dawn. They mate in particular seasons. Some species hibernate every winter, then return to activity. Birds and salmon migrate and return, almost like clockwork, according to the organizing intelligence of nature working within them.

Until recently, barely a hundred years out of millennia, human life, too, was organized in harmony with this profound intelligence. Today, with our concrete cities, our efficient technologies for heating, cooling, and lighting, our ability to ship food around the planet in hours, we tend to ignore these patterns.

But we are still intimately connected. Whether we consciously acknowledge it or not, we are part of the natural world. We are completely dependent upon the air we breathe, the water we drink, and the food we eat. Also, the biological rhythms of our own bodies are closely correlated with the rhythms that exist in nature. The changing of the seasons, the monthly 28-day circuit of the moon around the earth, the daily circadian cycle governed by the progress of the sun across the sky run steadily and irresistibly through our lives.

In a more natural state, people awaken with the sun and sleep when the moon is up, and somehow the body knows that. Even if you go to bed very late and remain asleep after the sun comes up, your body temperature, hormonal levels, and certain of your brain rhythms continue to rise and fall in tune with nature. For example, the level of cortisol, which helps your body handle stress, is high in the morning to help you prepare for the day's activities and drops in the evening as you relax toward sleep.

Because of this underlying correlation between the natural world and our human lives, it is helpful to learn how to take advantage of these cycles. Instead of living and acting in ways that ignore the natural tendencies of the body as it's being affected by the environment, it is health promoting to "go with the flow"—to align ourselves with nature's rhythms.

An Ideal Daily Routine

According to the ancient Ayurvedic sages, every day the earth passes through two cycles of Vata, Pitta, and Kapha:

First Cycle	Second Cycle
6 A.M. to 10 A.M. = Kapha	6 P.M. to 10 P.M. = Kapha
10 A.M. to 2 P.M. = Pitta	10 P.M. to 2 A.M. = Pitta
2 P.M. to 6 P.M. = Vata	2 A.M. to 6 A.M. = Vata

Ayurveda recommends a daily routine that corresponds with this recurring rhythm. This routine is preventive and at the same time promotes ideal mental and physical health.

The daily routine centers around four key times:

Rising 6 to 8 A.M.
Lunch Noon to 1 P.M.
Dinner 6 to 7 P.M.
Bedtime 9:30 to 10:30 P.M.

A day based around this schedule would look something like this:

Rising: 6 to 8 A.M.

Traditionally, Ayurveda recommends starting the day toward the end of the morning Vata period (around 5–6 A.M.), when lightness and clarity predominate and your mind and body have maximum chance for freshness. Since this is impractical for most of us, waking up between 6 and 8 is acceptable, but the longer you sleep into the Kapha period, the more you will tend to feel dull and heavy. Early rising is thus strongly recommended—before 6 if you can do it.

After rising:

- Drink a glass of warm water.
- Empty bladder and bowels (the warm water will help).
- Clean mouth and teeth; scrape tongue (special tongue scrapers are available at many natural food stores).
- Swish a little sesame oil in your mouth, discard, then rinse with warm water. This is traditionally said to prevent diseases of the gums and mouth. Alternately, you can lightly massage your gums with your finger and a little sesame oil.
- Massage your body with warm sesame oil (Abhyanga). (See illustrations and instructions on pages 58–60.)
- Bathe (warm water).
- Exercise according to your constitutional type. A good exercise program for all body types includes
  - "Salute to the Sun"—An invigorating stretching exercise. (See pages 99–101.)
  - Yoga Postures (pages 102–112).
  - Breathing Exercises (page 65).

- Meditation (pp. 66–71).
- Breakfast.

This sounds like a lot to do first thing in the morning, but if you try it for a few days, you'll probably feel so good you won't want to eliminate anything from this routine. At the least, it is recommended that you do a 1- to 2-minute "mini-massage" followed by a bath or shower, a few minutes of exercise, and a period of meditation.

After this morning routine, jump into several hours of focused activity, until lunchtime.

Lunch: Noon to 1 P.M.

Twelve o'clock is the height of Pitta, when appetite and "digestive fire" are at their peak. This is the time the digestive system is most efficient, so it is a good idea to eat your largest meal of the day now. Be sure to take enough time to eat sitting down, not reading, not watching TV, not opening mail. Eating on the run is a good way to compromise digestion and throw the entire system out of balance. Follow your meal with a short walk (5 to 15 miutes).

After lunch, resume your day's activities. The afternoon (2:00–6:00) is Vata time and is especially good for mental activities, whether work or study.

A second period of meditation in the late afternoon, between work and dinner, will help dissolve the stress of the day and give you more energy to enjoy the evening.

Dinner: 6 to 7 P.M.

Because the evening hours are dominated by Kapha, which is heavy and slow, it is best not to eat a lot at this time, since digestion will not be strong. Ayurveda recommends that dinner be a smaller meal than lunch, and that it be relatively easy to digest.

After dinner:

- Take a short walk (5 to 15 minutes) to promote digestion.
- Spend the evening pleasantly and quietly, reading, listening to music, or with friends and family. Avoid high-action movies or TV programs, as these are too stimulating as a prelude to sleep.

Bedtime: 9:30 to 10:30 P.M.

Since the Kapha phase of the daily cycle occurs in the evening, Kapha constitutional types naturally feel drowsy and by nature prefer going to bed early. However, Ayurveda recommends an early bedtime for everyone. This is to ensure that you get a full night of deep rest, which a number of research studies have correlated with optimum health and longevity.

If you are still up and about once the Pitta period begins at around 10 P.M., you will begin to feel more lively and alert; although you had been getting drowsy, you will suddenly feel more like reading, talking, or catching up on some letter writing or bill paying. Once this "second wind" kicks in and you start on these activities, you are liable to stay up quite late, and that is the end of your good night's rest.

The preceding guidelines are universal, and are beneficial for anyone of any constitutional type. However, as always in Ayurveda, there are certain constitution-specific suggestions that can be made.

For example, staying up late aggravates Vata. Bill, a former professional musician who was in the habit of staying up very late at night, was suffering from insomnia, worry, and difficulty in concentrating at his new job. When he had these problems earlier in his life, doctors had routinely prescribed Valium or some other tranquilizer or sleeping tablets. These helped him in the short run, but he couldn't take them for long, for fear of becoming dependent on them or suffering from the side effects.

Looking for a more natural alternative, Bill consulted a physician trained in Ayurvedic medicine.

"I have a very simple, very natural alternative for you," the doctor told him, "but it will require a real commitment from you." Bill said he was willing to try it.

"It's simply this: Go to bed at the same time every night, and make it before 10:30."

He didn't like the idea, but he wasn't happy with his insomnia and restlessness, either, or with the prospect of taking medications. Bill reorganized his life, and within a few weeks reported that from just this one adjustment he was sleeping more deeply and feeling much better.

Anyone who goes to bed late at night runs an increased risk of developing Vata disorders such as anxiety, insomnia, constipation, or high blood pressure. That's why it's good for all of us to go to bed reasonably early. But this guideline is particularly important for a Vata personality, who is constitutionally much more susceptible to Vata imbalance.

Similarly, skipping lunch is considered Pitta aggravating. High-energy Pitta types often think they're just too busy to stop for lunch, or they don't get around to eating until late in the day, but they're the ones who most need a noon lunch break.

Because noon is when the "digestive fire" burns brightest, it's important for Pittas to put something in the stomach at that time. Otherwise, the body tends to attack itself with digestive enzymes— to digest itself, so to speak. As a result, problems such as ulcers (generally a Pitta disorder) can develop. Psychologically, anger and aggressive tendencies, which are caused by Pitta, can be exacerbated by skipping lunch; these problems can often be soothed and balanced simply by eating a good-sized meal around noon.

Sleeping in the daytime increases Kapha. It is quite possible to aggravate or even bring on a cold, nasal or bronchial congestion, sinus troubles, or certain types of arthritis just by sleeping in the daytime. Depression, which is frequently caused by excess Kapha, is commonly intensified by daytime sleep. So, especially if you have a tendency toward lethargy or laziness, try to wake up early and get going.

Here are two more suggestions for a nature-based routine, useful for all constitutional types.

- Most people have their biggest meal at supper, only a few hours before going to bed. This is a common cause for colds, congestion, stomach aches, insomnia, and acid stomach. Instead of reaching for an antacid, restructure your schedule. Have your main meal early; eat lightly at night. You might try cooked cereal and toast, or rice or another light grain with some vegetables. It is best to avoid meat, yogurt, and cheese especially in your evening meal.

- If you enjoy sports, the best time is during the two Kapha periods of the day, particularly in the morning (6–10 A.M.). Exercise helps to balance Kapha; it reduces sluggishness, congestion, and lethargy, and it brings vitality to the whole physiology.

Following a good daily routine is important as a preventive measure and in the treatment of many illnesses, since according to Ayurveda many illnesses are generated or worsened just by being out of synch with nature's rhythms. Just a few changes in lifestyle—getting up earlier, eating less at night, going to bed on time—can go a long way toward alleviating a condition that otherwise might have to be treated by powerful drugs or other drastic measures later on.

A good daily routine, consisting of the elements we know are health building for our constitutional type, is a master key to good health and emotional well-being. As David Frawley writes in his book *Ayurvedic Healing,*

> There is no substitute for our own right living. It cannot be bought at any price and we cannot expect another to provide it. As long as we are not living in harmony with our nature and constitution we cannot expect ourselves to be really healed by any method.
>
> It is the beauty of Ayurveda that it gives each of us the knowledge and means to live in harmony. It provides us with the right regime for our particular type, covering all aspects of our nature, physical, psychological, and spiritual. But it can only succeed with our own time and effort, devotion and dedication.
>
> What we do every day is our real religion, for it shows what we truly value in life. . . . What we do every day makes for who we are.

Health for All Seasons

Another key to maintaining good health and preventing illness is to understand and respond to the changes of seasons. As the weather changes, our minds and bodies also go through transformations. If we ignore this influence and act as if we were somehow exempt from the powerful forces of nature, we'll have to pay the penalty.

In the Ayurvedic scheme of things, there are three main seasons, corresponding to the three main body types.

Vata season
Vata season covers fall and winter. Depending on where you live, you will find it lasting from around October/November to February/March. The exact timing will vary according to your location (it comes earlier and lasts longer in the Midwest, for example,

compared to its duration in California or Florida). During Vata season, the Vata qualities—cold, windy, dry, light—are in ascendance.

Kapha season

Kapha season corresponds to spring. Lasting approximately from February until May, Kapha season is wet and cool.

Pitta season

Pitta season is summertime. It is hot, often humid, and lasts from around June through September.

With this in mind, let's take a ride through the seasons, noting what we can do to maintain good health the year round.

Tips for Optimum Health in Spring Season (March–May)

The qualities of Kapha season are heavy, cold, sticky, slow, and moist. In our bodies, Kapha governs our physical structure and fluid balance. If you keep these points in mind it will be easy to understand the kinds of problems that can crop up when the influence of Kapha increases in nature during Kapha season.

Rosemary has never been fond of spring. As lovely as it was to see the flowers and buds on the trees, she has never really been able to enjoy it. It seemed that every spring, without fail, she would have a cold and mucous congestion in her sinuses, ending up with bronchitis or at least a lingering cough. As she got older, she also began to experience joint pain and attacks of arthritis, due to a thickening of the synovial fluid (which lubricates the joints).

If that weren't enough, she felt a kind of heaviness and mental dullness that sometimes slipped into depression. Her motivation and ambition dropped, and she felt tired and lethargic for days on end. With those qualities dominating, it was far too easy for her to put on weight.

These tendencies affect everyone during the spring season, but they are much more likely to trouble you if, like Rosemary, you have a Kapha constitution. Every year, as Kapha increases in nature, it increases in us, too.

Rosemary always thought she had a kind of curse, which her husband Bob had miraculously escaped. A wiry Vata type, Bob always felt energetic and enlivened as spring approached. This is because Vata is in most respects directly opposite to Kapha, so just when Kaphas start to feel stuffed up and bogged down, Vatas tend to feel most balanced and happy.

When Rosemary began to follow the recommendations I will share with you in a moment, her whole experience of spring changed for the better.

Since anyone can accumulate excess Kapha and thus develop an imbalance in Kapha season, it is helpful to learn how to keep this heavy, sluggish tendency from increasing too much in us. Then we can enjoy the positive qualities of *balanced* Kapha: happiness, strength, kindness, compassion, generosity, loyalty, good memory, strong immunity, a love of romance, and wholeness of consciousness.

Stoke your digestive fire

Digestion tends to become sluggish during the spring; you can perk it up by following these suggestions:

- Eat hot food—both hot in temperature and spicy.
- Drink hot, stimulating drinks, such as fresh ginger tea.
- Cut down on refined sugars. Substitute raw, unheated honey, which is very effective in reducing Kapha.
- Favor foods that taste astringent (such as lentils and beans), spicy (chile peppers or curries, for example), and bitter (salads, spinach).
- Eat a ginger pickle before lunch or dinner to help increase your "digestive fire." To make a ginger pickle, sprinkle lemon juice and salt on a thin slice of fresh ginger. (Alternatively, you can grate the ginger and mix with lemon and salt.) Eat about 15 minutes before a meal.
- Sip hot water frequently during the day. This is also an excellent preventative and treatment for colds and sore throats.

Rise and shine

As mentioned earlier, a good way to combat the Kapha tendency toward dullness, lethargy, and depression is to get up early in the morning. If you get out of bed before 6:00 P.M., during Vata time, you will feel the benefit of the Vata lightness, clarity, and liveliness. The longer you stay in bed after 6:00, the more you will feel sluggish and tired. To help you get up early, go to bed during the evening Kapha time, before 10:00 P.M., when you begin to feel drowsy. Then you'll sleep deeply and wake up naturally with the sun.

Get more exercise

To keep from putting on weight or giving in to the blues during Kapha season, it helps to get some extra exercise, especially for people with a Kapha constitution. The best times for exercise are 6:00 to 10:00 A.M., and 6:00 to 8:00 P.M. After the frozen winter, everybody really needs to move, and this is what nature expresses, too, with spring's burst of energy and growth.

Stay Balanced in the Summer (June–September)

As the days lengthen and the sun rises in the sky, spring's cool, moist Kapha qualities burn off, giving way to the heat of summer. Because the connection between ourselves and our environment is so strong, all aspects of mind and body are influenced by the increase in temperature. This can have a positive or a negative effect, depending upon our constitutional type and whether we're able to harness the positive qualities of increased Pitta without getting out of balance.

If too much Pitta accumulates in our system—especially likely in a person with a Pitta body type—we may develop skin inflammations, acid stomach, burning sensations in the body, red eyes, and moles and freckles on the skin. Any tendency toward graying hair or balding will be accelerated. And tempers can flare as anger and irritation rise with the temperatures.

On the other hand, if Pitta grows stronger but remains balanced, you may notice increased focus and mental clarity, spontaneous feelings of joyfulness, and increased energy, vitality, and strength.

To keep cool and promote the highest quality of experience during Pitta season, pay attention to the following guidelines.

- *Lighten up.* Enjoy light entertainment such as comedies, joke telling, walks in the garden or the woods, and playing with children.
- *Calm down with meditation.* Practice meditation to lower your mental temperature. Meditation decreases stress and agitation

and produces a calming influence that leaves you feeling refreshed.

- *Cool down anger with awareness.* If you become angry, try to be
  aware that "this is only the result of some imbalance of Pitta in
  my body." Remaining as objective as possible, you can take
  steps to balance the situation, including most of the suggestions
  in this list. Start by drinking a glass of cold water. If someone you
  know suffers from Pitta attacks, try not to take the anger personally; do what you can to help them cool down.

- *Watch your diet.* Eat a Pitta-pacifying diet. Choose cooler food
  and drinks. Favor foods with these three tastes:
  - bitter (salads, green leafy vegetables)
  - sweet (dairy, rice, clarified butter, sweet fruits)
  - astringent (lentils, beans).

  Stay away from salty, sour, and spicy foods. Save those Mexican dinners for the winter season.

- *Go to the herb garden.* Use Pitta-pacifying herbs such as fennel,
  coriander, cumin, and cardamom in cooking and teas. Chewing on fennel seeds from time to time during the day (they
  taste sweet and a lot like licorice) is very cooling.

- *Don't overdo it.* Keep exercise moderate and aim for the cooler
  early morning hours, or the early evening. Water exercise and
  sports (swimming, water polo) are especially cooling. Pitta types
  especially must be careful not to overexercise in Pitta season or
  participate in sports in the middle of a hot summer afternoon.

- *Try a cooling, calming massage.* A 5-minute daily self-massage
  with coconut oil prior to bathing is very pacifying to Pitta and
  will help maintain emotional balance throughout the day.

- *Use cooling fragrances.* Among these are jasmine and rose,
  which are relaxing to mind and body during the hot summer.
  These are available as aromatic oils and incense; you don't
  need much to produce a nice effect.

- *Surround yourself with beauty.* Try to spend some time in a
  beautiful flower garden or near a fountain—these are very
  soothing to Pittas.

- *Listen to peaceful music.* Certain music can calm mind and
  body and lower mental-emotional temperatures. Classical Indian music or the slow movements of classical music (particularly the regular rhythms of Baroque composers such as Bach,

Handel, and Telemann) produce a calming effect. (This is also very useful for high-strung Vata types at any time of year.)

Following these recommendations for Pitta season will help you enjoy your summer without boiling over.

Keep Healthy and Happy in Autumn and Winter (October–February)

Vata season, with its light, dry, cold qualities, tends to increase Vata tendencies in our mental and physical makeup. Positive Vata qualities such as enthusiasm, energy, lightheartedness, and creativity increase in us so long as we maintain balance. If Vata increases too much and becomes aggravated, we may fall victim to anxiety, insomnia, dry skin, constipation, or difficulty with memory and concentration. Rapid heartbeat, high blood pressure, and a tendency toward an erratic schedule are more of the negative effects of aggravated Vata. Although Vata individuals are especially prone to these imbalances, everyone can benefit from knowing how to pacify or calm Vata to maintain health and balance during the fall season.

Stay on schedule
Probably the single most important thing you can do to keep Vata in balance is to maintain a regular daily routine. Unfortunately, for people of a Vata nature this can be quite difficult, as Vatas are often the kind of people whose "schedules" are different every day. But irregular daily habits tend to adversely affect the nervous system, which is controlled by Vata, so it is helpful to wake up, exercise, meditate, eat, and go to bed at approximately the same times every day.

Go to bed early
Staying up late is one of the major factors that increase Vata, so try to be in bed between the hours of 9:00 and 10:30.

Eat three squares a day
Missing meals is also very imbalancing. The noon meal should be the largest meal of the day. Breakfast is optional, especially for Kapha types, but is recommended for Vatas, who need a solid, grounding meal such as cereal, toast, and milk to combat the Vata tendency toward spaciness. Dinner should be on the lighter side.

Eight More Tips for Keeping Vata in Balance

1. To reduce the likelihood of insomnia, restrict your activities in the evening to the lighter side. Don't do any concentrated work and avoid fast-paced, stimulating movies or TV programs. Some pleasant reading or listening to soft music are ideal.

2. Practice meditation to relax and reduce anxiety, stress, and tension. A successful meditation technique allows the mind to become very still, much as a choppy lake can become settled and silent. Due to the interconnectedness of mind and body, the physiology also becomes relaxed when the mind quiets down.

3. Follow a Vata-pacifying diet. Favor warm food and drinks and eat more oily foods such as nuts, or vegetables with butter or ghee. Lean toward foods with predominantly sweet, sour, and salty tastes; reduce or avoid foods that are light, dry, or cold.

4. Unless prescribed by your doctor, Vata season is not the time for fasting or an unusually light diet, such as salads or a lot of raw foods. Well-cooked, heavier foods are better in this season.

5. Some herbs that you can use to help balance Vata are cinnamon, ginger, cumin, fenugreek, and asafoetida (*hing*). The Indian herbs *ashvagandha* and *bala* are excellent for balancing Vata.

6. A warm sesame oil self-massage each morning prior to bathing is particularly helpful in promoting emotional stability and mental clarity throughout the day. If you have trouble sleeping, massage the soles of your feet with warm sesame oil for a few minutes before getting into bed.

7. Keep warm. Wear a hat to protect your head and stay out of the wind as much as you can.

8. Regular exercise is helpful, but not to extremes, especially if you have a Vata constitution. It is best not to exercise outdoors during Vata season; the dry, cold air can cause respiratory problems and aggravate Vata.

Do your best to incorporate these seasonal guidelines into your life. They will help you to avoid potential health problems and to enjoy the positive qualities that naturally get enlivened with each change of the seasons.

CHAPTER 7

CREATING YOUR PERSONAL BODY-TYPE EXERCISE PLAN

From an Ayurvedic perspective, the purpose of exercise is to re-duce stress, cleanse our body of toxins, improve circulation and di-gestion, and tone and rejuvenate the whole system. It should also develop coordination between mind and body, so the two can work together to create perfect health. Charaka, one of the great ancient exponents of Ayurveda, said that "from physical exercise one gets lightness, a capacity for work, firmness, tolerance of diffi-culties, elimination of impurities, and stimulation of digestion."

You can see how far away our current exercise theories and practices are from this balanced approach. Body building and in-tensive aerobic workouts may be good for some people, but as a general standard for optimum health they leave much to be desired.

In this chapter you will learn a series of exercises that are good for all body types. You'll also learn how to develop an exer-cise program ideally suited for your own particular constitution. And you will acquire some key principles that will help you enjoy your exercise much more and get much more out of it.

But first, in case you are a person who does little or no physical exercise, don't despair—you are not alone. The vast majority of Americans are in your camp. Research repeatedly shows that fewer than 15 percent of Americans engage in a regular exercise program.

I don't want to scare you (maybe just motivate you a little) but the results of our passivity are disastrous. An inactive body loses flexibility, muscle strength, and aerobic capacity. People who are sedentary are at greater risk for many diseases, such as diabetes, hypertension, colon and breast cancers, and osteoporosis.

The greatest risk is for heart disease, the nation's number-one killer. Just recently, the American Heart Association added physical inactivity to its list of major risk factors for heart disease.

The good news is that only a modest increase in our exercise level can be extremely beneficial. And since the amount we exercise is largely within our control, we can greatly improve our health by making a simple change in our lifestyle.

What Exercise Can Do for Your Health

An appropriate exercise program helps your body maintain strong immunity, normal blood sugar levels, and healthy brain chemistry. Sufficient exercise is an important factor in deep, restful sleep and can be helpful in warding off depression. It's a key factor in keeping the digestive system strong and not sluggish, so we can get full nourishment from the food we eat.

Exercise also strengthens the heart and cardiovascular system, bringing such gains as increased cardiac efficiency (more blood pumped by each heartbeat), a slower pulse, decreased workload on the heart, lower blood pressure, less tendency for blood clots to form, decreased chance of degeneration of the arteries, and lower overall cholesterol along with higher "good" HDL cholesterol.

People who exercise all their lives, not just when they're young, will be able to retain a full measure of physical strength and stamina into old age. This is one of the major findings of recent aging studies, which suggest that the body does not necessarily have to decline or "wear out" as it gets older. What's more, people who exercise using Ayurvedic principles and practices will gain energy, flexibility, and joyfulness as well as better strength and more robust health.

Three Keys to Getting the Most From Exercise

All right, then, exercise is crucial for good health. But how much do we really need? And what kind? Here are three Ayurvedic principles to help you derive maximum benefit from your exercise.

Enjoy your exercise

The main reason most of us don't exercise is not that we are, deep down, nothing but lazy, good-for-nothing couch potatoes—!—but simply that we have rarely found exercise to be enjoyable. We've all been brought up believing that exercise has to be difficult to be worthwhile; we've had gym coaches blowing whistles and shouting commands at us like Marine sergeants, we've pushed our bodies beyond what they could comfortably do, embarrassed ourselves trying to play sports we had no particular aptitude for—and as a result, exercise has little appeal.

Ayurveda says that exercise should be enjoyable, suited to our nature, and always within our comfort zone. Pushing oneself to perform is fine for a highly trained competitive athlete, but for the rest of us, it creates strain on the body that leads to stress, weakness, and more rapid aging.

Don't strain—take it easy!

Despite all the hoopla over the importance of vigorous aerobic exercise, several key studies involving thousands of participants have shown that moderate exercise such as walking, gardening, and home repair produced virtually the same benefits as high-intensity exercise. In one study of more than 13,000 men and women, the greatest health gains were in the group who simply walked for 30 minutes a day.

This finding precisely matches the age-old advice of the Ayurvedic tradition. According to Ayurveda, moderate exercise is not only sufficient, it is the most beneficial. Contrary to the prevailing "no pain, no gain" philosophy, any exercise that causes discomfort or strain is considered harmful. To be most effective, exercise should be easy, enjoyable, and suited to your body type.

Learning to judge how much exercise is enough is an important skill. Not only does it differ from person to person, but it will differ for you on different days. There may be days when you can

HOW TO DETERMINE YOUR OPTIMUM EXERCISE HEART RATE

The Formula:

$$\frac{220 - \text{your age} + \text{your resting heart rate}}{2}$$

Example 1: For a 40-year-old with a resting heart rate of 70 beats per minute.

$$220 - 40 = 180$$
$$180 + 70 = 250$$
$$250/2 = 125$$

Your maximum heart rate during exercise should be about 125 beats per minute.

Example 2: For a 60 year old with a resting heart rate of 60 beats per minute.

$$220 - 60 = 160$$
$$160 + 60 = 220$$
$$220/2 = 110$$

Your maximum heart rate during exercise should be about 110 beats per minute.

Note: If you have had an exercise stress test (treadmill), use the maximum heart rate from your test instead of 220.

---

push yourself a little harder and enjoy it, and days when you need to take it easy. You can use the knowledge of your optimum heart rate (see above) as a baseline guide, but it is also good to learn to judge subjectively how it feels when you are exercising at your top level and how you feel when you pass that level and begin to strain.

Listen to your body

Dr. John Douillard, author of *Body, Mind and Sport* (up to now the only complete exercise and fitness book based on the principles of Ayurveda) suggests that we learn to "listen" carefully to our bodies during exercise, in order to recognize what he calls the "breaking point": that point at which we begin to feel some discomfort or strain. His studies show that this comes when we reach about 50 percent of our capacity. Going beyond this causes undue strain and gives your body extra repair work to do.

If you break out in a heavy sweat; if you lose the feeling of comfort; if your heart starts pounding strongly; or if you start panting, have difficulty breathing, or feel you need to breathe through your mouth—you're working too hard. When this happens, cut back. Slow down. Wait until your body feels comfortable again, then gradually pick up the pace, "listening" carefully to how your body feels. This is another example of self-referral, the process of tuning in to yourself described in Chapter 3.

Don't forget to apply these principles to the exercise recommendations that follow in the rest of the chapter.

Three Exercises for Everybody

Ayurvedic treatments and recommendations for healthy living are based on individual differences. That's why the kinds of exercises and the degree of exertion recommended for different body types are different. Later in this chapter I'll suggest a number of exercises and sports that are the most appropriate for *your* constitution. Three exercises, however, are prescribed for all body types and all ages.

Walking

A brisk walk every day, for about half an hour, preferably in the fresh early-morning air, is considered an ideal exercise for everyone. Walking provides nearly as much benefit to the heart as other exercises requiring greater exertion, *and it is far safer.* (The number of exercise-related cardiac incidents is far smaller from walking than from running or racquetball!)

Try to take your walk between 6 A.M. and 10 A.M., during the Kapha time of day. The earlier the better. This is the ideal time for all exercise, and for all body types. Second best is the evening Kapha period (6 to 10 P.M.) but try to finish by 8 o'clock so you don't get your system running in high gear too close to bedtime.

If it isn't practical for you to go out for a walk before you meditate and eat breakfast, then how about walking to work? Or parking far enough away from your workplace so you can get in a good walk on the way to work, and another one afterwards? Maybe you can use part of your lunch break, or you can walk for a while after dinner. If possible, take your walk in a beautiful natural setting.

If you feel you are too busy to go outdoors every day (weather permitting, of course) to appreciate the beauty of nature, with the sun on your face and the cool touch of the breeze, then you *are* too busy. These influences are some of the best and most powerful medicines you can get. A walk through the fresh air of early morning brings the senses alive and makes the body and mind feel lively and awake in a way that no exercise machine possibly can.

Salutation to the sun

The second universally recommended exercise is known as the Salutation to the Sun. This is an easy, graceful exercise that stretches the body and also helps the mind to become calm. A series of 12 Yoga poses that flow into one another without a break, the Sun Salutation helps to integrate mind, body, and breath.

The Sun Salutation is, by itself, a complete exercise, and its benefits have been extolled in the Ayurvedic texts for thousands of years. As the muscles of the body are flexed during the 12 postures, the internal organs are also massaged, and the spine goes through a wide range of motion, increasing flexibility and releasing tension.

A good pace for this exercise is to take about 5 seconds to perform each posture, adding up to a total of about 1 minute for a complete cycle. You can go through the sequence more slowly for

BENEFITS OF THE SUN SALUTATION

- Improves circulation, energy, and vitality
- Massages the internal organs
- Increases flexibility of the spine
- Releases tightness in the rib cage, which inhibits deep breathing
- Sends energy into every cell of the body
- Increases muscle strength and flexibility

Best of all, performing Sun Salutations feels really good!

Note: Points on the benefits of the Salutation to the Sun are adapted from *Body, Mind and Sport* by John Douillard (Harmony Books, 1994).

stretching and relaxation, or more quickly for a good aerobic workout. Anywhere from 5 to 10 cycles is recommended, but you should start with only 1 or 2, especially if you are over 40 or if this is the first exercise you are doing in a long time.

While doing the Sun Salutation, be sure to follow the directions for breathing given with each posture. Breathe in when stretching or extending, and out when bending or contracting. Throughout the exercise, breathe somewhat deeply, through the nose.

In each posture, stretch only as far as you are comfortable. If you feel some pain or tension developing, don't push it. Soon you'll find yourself stretching way beyond what limited you before.

Once you learn the individual postures, perform the whole series together without a break. The postures should flow into one another in a smooth, fluid flow.

For results that go beyond physical conditioning, perform the Salutation to the Sun with conscious attention. If your mind is off somewhere else, then you will reap only minimal benefits and relatively no integration of mind and body, which is one of the most important benefits of exercise. If you keep your awareness on what you're doing, your mind will become settled and quiet. This is true of any exercise you do. To heighten this experience of inner quietness, do the postures more slowly.

Please note: This exercise is not recommended during pregnancy. It may also pose problems for orthopedic patients; if this pertains to you, consult your doctor about it.

The Postures

1. **Salutation Position**   (Inhale and exhale)
   Remember: All breathing should be through your nose.

   Stand erect with your feet together and your weight evenly on both feet. Hold the palms of your hands together in front of your chest and look straight ahead.

2. **Raised Arm Position**   (Inhale)

   Inhale while slowly extending your arms above your head. Reach up and slightly back, allowing your eyes to look upward.

3. **Hand to Foot Position**   (Exhale)

As you exhale, bend forward and down. Keep your knees straight *only if it's comfortable for you.* Otherwise, let them bend freely as you bring your hands to the floor. Keep elbows and shoulders relaxed. If you can't comfortably touch the floor, that's fine. Just go as far as is comfortable.

4. Equestrian Position (Inhale)

Extend your right leg back and drop the knee to the ground. The left (front) knee is bent, foot flat on the floor. Lengthen your spine and expand your chest as you stretch your head and neck comfortably upward.

5. Mountain Position (Exhale)

Bring your left leg back to meet the right leg. Keep hands and feet at shoulder distance apart. Raise your buttocks and hips, pressing down with your hands. If you can, press your heels down toward the floor. Relax your head and neck.

6. Eight Limbs Position (Hold breath briefly)

Slowly drop both knees to the ground and ease down until eight points on your body—both feet, knees, and hands, as well as chest and chin—touch the floor. Hold very briefly before gliding into the next pose.

7. Cobra Position (Inhale)

Pull your chest up, using your back muscles. Don't push up with your arms or pull up from your head or neck. Keep your elbows close to the body as you extend the spine upward.

8. Mountain Position (Exhale)

Repeat position 5.

9. Equestrian Position (Inhale)

Repeat position 4 with right leg forward this time.

10. Hand to Foot Position (Exhale)

Repeat position 3.

11. Raised Arm Position (Inhale)

Repeat position 2.

12. Salutation Position (Exhale)

Repeat position 1.

If you are continuing to another cycle, you can breathe in and out slowly a few times to get centered, or just exhale and continue on, as you feel.

Simple Yoga Postures for All Body Types

The following yoga postures are good for all constitutional types. Anyone, of any age, can practice them, so long as you are in good health and don't strain yourself trying to do a posture perfectly. If you have any health problems, especially of a musculoskeletal nature, you should consult with a physician before doing these exercises. Also, yoga exercises should be avoided during pregnancy, especially the last 5–6 months.

These *asanas* (postures, positions) are part of any Ayurvedic health program. They promote flexibility, strength, and vitality and give an inner massage to the body's vital organs that increases circulation and blood flow. They are excellent for improving health.

Take some time to learn them at the outset, so you can do them effortlessly and correctly without referring to the pictures and descriptions. Once you get to the stage where you don't have to think about them, you will find them enjoyable and relaxing to perform.

Here are some points to make your practice of these postures most comfortable and beneficial:

Never strain

This is the key rule for yoga postures. Don't try to make the posture "picture perfect." Just bend or stretch as far as you can without pain. It's okay to feel a little pull or stretch, but stop at that point. Over a few weeks or months, your flexibility will gradually increase if you do these postures regularly.

Don't force it

These are not like gym-class calisthenics, so don't "bounce" your body to get into the position. Just stretch until you feel you've gone as far as you comfortably can, hold for a few seconds, and release.

Never feel like you have to look like the picture. The picture is the "ideal posture," but ideal for you is whatever is comfortable without straining.

- Your movements should be slow, never abrupt.
- Breathe normally at all times.
- It's better not to have music or any other distraction (radio, TV) while you're doing these postures. In fact, it is helpful to allow your awareness to be on the body as you move through the postures. Be with what you're doing.

- Wear loose, comfortable clothing that doesn't impede your movements.

- Don't do the postures on a bare floor. Use an exercise mat or a folded blanket (wool or cotton is best). Your mat should be firm enough for support, not too soft.

- Do the postures in the sequence given here. Each pose is a preparation for the next or a counterbalance—a forward bend after a backward bend, etc.

- Wait at least 1-1/2 hours after a snack, 3–4 hours after a full meal before doing yoga postures. Also, wait about half an hour after completing the postures before eating.

- A recommended time is mentioned in parentheses for each posture. This is an approximate time, not an exact time, and may be too long for your comfort at first. You may need to start with just a few seconds for each posture, then gradually increase. Again, *comfort* is the main principle.

- After completing each posture, *rest* for a few moments before moving on to the next pose. The exception to this is that you can go directly from the shoulder stand into the plow pose without a rest. (See below.)

One set of these postures will take you about 15 minutes to complete. However, if you've never done yoga postures before, you will probably need longer the first few times as you learn the positions.

Toning up (1 to 2 minutes)
This is a warm-up for the whole body, to increase circulation and prepare for the other postures.

1. Sit comfortably and use your palms and fingers to give a massage to the whole body. Starting with the top of your head, press firmly (but gently) with both hands, release, move your hands an inch or so forward, press, release, move forward . . . and continue pressing and letting up as you move over your face and down the neck to your chest. Remember to use both palms and fingers. Use this press-and-release movement for the entire toning up. (Don't just slide your hands; press and release.)

Starting again at the top of your head, press and release as you move your hands to the back of your head and neck and come around your shoulders to your chest.

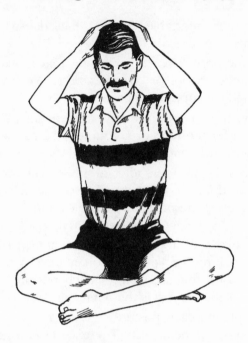

2. Next do your arms. With your left hand, grasp the fingers of your right hand and press and release as you move up the top of your arm, from hand to forearm to shoulder and across to your chest. Repeat with the bottom of your arm, then do your left hand and arm with your right hand.

3. With fingertips at your navel and palms on your abdomen, press and release as you move gradually up toward your heart.

4. Reach around to your lower back and press and release as you move your hands up and around your ribs again toward the heart.

5. Massage your right foot, starting with the toes and moving up to your ankle, calf, thigh, and hip as you press and release up to the chest. Repeat with your left foot and leg, pressing and releasing with palms and fingers up toward the heart.

6. Lie on your back. Bring your knees to your chest, grasp your knees, and roll slowly from side to side 5 or 6 times. Allow your head and neck to move freely.

7. Lie on your back with legs outstretched and relax.

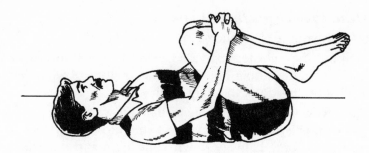

Seat-firming posture (30 seconds)

1. Kneel with your feet slightly apart and big toes crossed. Drop down until you're sitting on your feet, buttocks on your ankles and heels. Place your hands in your lap, palms up, right hand on top. Hold your head high and your back straight.

2. Lift up into a kneeling position, keeping your spine straight, shoulders relaxed (not pulled up). Inhale as you rise up, and then exhale as you sit back down. Repeat once or twice, moving slowly.

Benefits: This posture strengthens the knees, ankles, and legs and the pelvic region and is good for the back. It is said to relieve gas and to aid digestion if it is done right after eating. (This is an exception to the rule of not performing the asanas immediately after meals.)

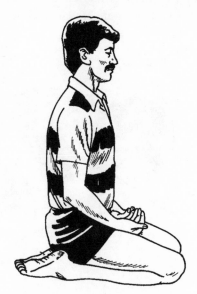

Head-to-knee posture (1 minute)

1. Sit with your legs extended in front of you.

2. Keeping the right leg extended, bend your left leg (with your knee near the floor) and bring the bottom of your left foot against the inside of the right thigh.

3. Bend forward, with arms outstretched toward the right foot. If you can, grasp the toes, but don't strain to do so. Your fingers may reach only halfway down your leg, or to the ankle, and that's fine. Keep your right leg straight if you can, otherwise you may bend it slightly. Hold for 10 to 15 seconds, come up slowly, and repeat on the same side.

4. Now repeat the position, this time with the left leg extended. Do the posture twice, each time holding for about 10 to 15 seconds.

5. It's good to exhale as you bend forward and inhale as you straighten up.

Note: If you are experienced with yoga postures, instead of stretching toward one foot at a time, you can do this pose with both feet together, bending forward comfortably and grasping the toes. You can hold the pose for up to 30 seconds. But remember—*don't strain!*

Benefits: This postures stretches and relaxes the spine and tones the organs of the abdomen. It also facilitates elimination.

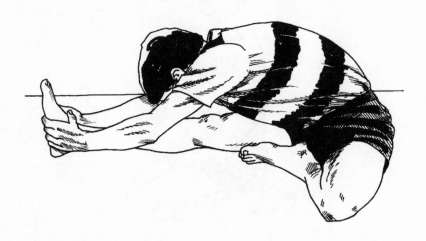

Shoulder stand (start with 30 seconds; can gradually increase to 2 minutes if comfortable)

1. Lie flat on your back, hands at your sides.

2. Raise your legs slowly, then, supporting your back with your hands, raise legs and trunk all the way to a vertical position, until your chin presses against your chest. In the half shoulder stand, the body is not completely straight as it is in the full shoulder stand. (See illustration.)

3. *Important:* Be careful not to place much weight or pressure on the neck or throat. This is a *shoulder* stand.

4. To come down, lower the legs slightly behind the head, replace your forearms on the floor, and gradually bring trunk and then legs back to the floor. Don't raise your head until your legs are back on the floor.

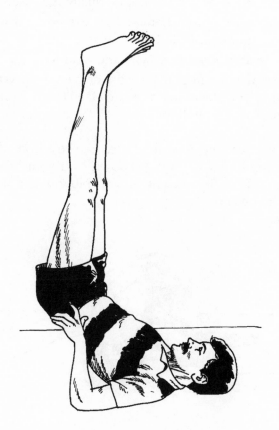

Note: If you are a beginner, do the *half shoulder stand* (p. 107) for several months until you are completely comfortable with it; then move to the full shoulder stand.

Benefits: This posture stimulates the thyroid gland and relieves physical and mental fatigue. It improves flexibility of the spine and is said to help with asthma, disorders of the liver and intestines, and heart trouble. Its name in Sanskrit is *sarvangasana,* which means a posture beneficial for the whole body.

Plow posture (15 seconds to 1 minute)

1. Lie flat on your back with hands alongside the body, palms down. Press your palms to the floor and raise your legs, then your hips and lower back, continuing to move your legs back behind your head.

2. Bring your feet back only so far as they are comfortable. They may not touch the floor at first. If you feel strain, come back out of the pose. Flexibility will gradually increase.

3. With toes on the floor behind you, extend your arms out opposite to your feet. Hold for a few seconds.

4. Fold your arms over your head and hold for a few seconds.

5. To come down, support your lower back with your hands as you bring your feet back forward. Don't raise your head until legs are back on the floor.

Note: You can go into this pose directly from the shoulder stand by slowly bringing your legs down over your head until your feet touch the floor. Shoulder stand and plow would then be done in one continuous flow.

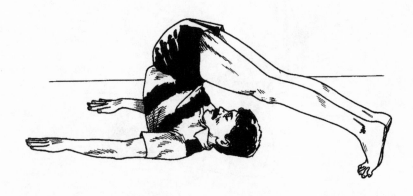

Benefits: Like the shoulder stand, the plow stimulates the all-important thyroid gland. It strengthens the back and is excellent for increasing flexibility of the spine. The plow pose is helpful for the liver and spleen and aids in normalizing digestion and elimination.

Cobra posture (30 seconds to 1 minute)

1. Lie face down, feet together and hands under your shoulders, palms down, toes pointed backward.
2. Slowly lift your head, neck, and chest as far as you can without straining. Although you will have to press down somewhat with your hands, this is *not* a push-up—rather, try to lift your chest with the help of the back muscles and use the hands mostly for support.
3. Hold for 10–15 seconds and come down slowly, lowering your trunk first, then your head.
4. Repeat 1 to 3 times.

Benefits: The cobra pose strengthens the back, expands the chest, and helps the spine be flexible. The posture is good for the abdominal muscles and helps relieve constipation and gas. It is also very helpful for uterine and ovarian health.

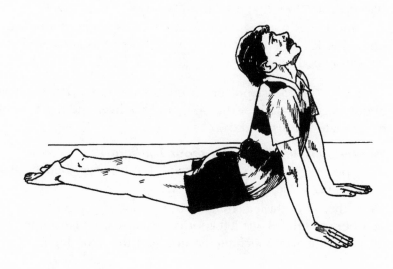

Locust posture (30 seconds to 1 minute)

1. Continue to lie face down (following the cobra pose). Keep your legs together, arms stretched back by your sides, palms up, chin resting on the floor.

2. Raise both legs upward, keeping the legs fully extended and the knees straight. Your full weight rests on your chest and arms.

3. Hold for a few seconds, then allow the legs to come down slowly. Repeat 1 to 3 times.

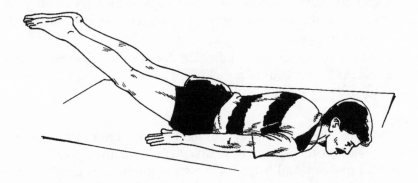

Note: This posture is not easy at first. Beginners can make it more comfortable in two ways:

1. Place hands under your thighs instead of at your sides.

2. Lift and lower one leg, repeat 1 to 3 times, then lift and lower the other leg and repeat 1 to 3 times. When this is comfortable, try lifting both legs at once.

Benefits: The locust posture exercises the lower back, pelvis, and abdomen. It is good for digestion and the liver and has benefits for the prostate, uterus, and ovaries.

Seated twisting posture (about 1 minute)

This posture is slightly complicated, but it is very beneficial so it's worth taking some time to master it.

1. Sit with your right leg straight out in front of you and your left leg bent, so that your left foot is next to your right knee, the inside of the foot touching the inside of the right thigh.

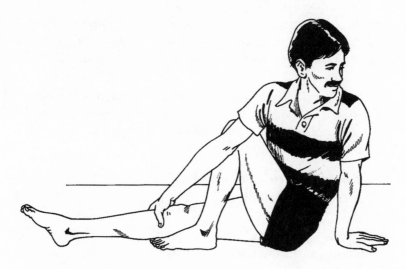

2. Do the following steps in one gradual motion as you twist *slowly* to the left:
  • Place your left hand on the floor behind you.
  • Reach your right hand around *outside* your left knee and grasp right knee (if you can).
  • Turn your head all the way to the left.
  • Bring your left hand up and around behind you.
3. Hold for a few seconds. Slowly come out of the pose by first turning your head back to center, the rest of the body following.
4. Repeat on the other side.

Benefits: This posture increases circulation to the abdominal organs, so it is beneficial for the liver, spleen, kidneys, and adrenals. It strengthens and relaxes the neck and back.

Standing forward bend (30 seconds to 1 minute)
1. Stand erect with feet slightly apart.
2. Raise your arms above your head, palms facing forward.
3. Bend forward and down. Keep your knees straight if you can, otherwise let them bend slightly as your hands approach the floor. Grasp your toes and bring your head in close to your knees, but *without strain*.

4. Hold for a few seconds, then come up the same way as you bent forward, lifting your arms above your head as you straighten up, then bringing them down to your sides.

Benefits: The forward bend nourishes the organs of the head due to increased blood supply. It tones the abdominal organs (kidneys, stomach, spleen, liver) and exercises the spine. It has a calming effect and is soothing to tired eyes.

Rest posture (1 to 2 minutes)

1. Lie on your back with legs slightly apart and arms loosely by your sides, palms up.
2. Close your eyes, relax, and lie quietly for a minute or two. When you are finished, *get up slowly.*

Benefits: The rest posture refreshes and invigorates the body.

Exercises for Your Body Type

Now we come to some suggestions specifically for you. Just as it is vital to eat foods that bring balance to your individual constitution, so it is also important to choose exercises that are appropriate for you. As spicy, oily, or even sweet foods are good for some people but not for others, so certain sports and exercises are beneficial to some of us but may actually be harmful to others.

For example, John, a 43-year-old ex-football player, still likes to run 4 miles a day, followed by an intensive weight-lifting session. He just can't understand why Larry, his 15-year-old son, doesn't like running, football, or weight lifting. Larry prefers hiking and camping with friends for recreation. He feels like a disappointment to his dad, but on the other hand is quite happy with his exercise preferences. What's the explanation?

The answer lies in the Ayurvedic body types. John has a strong, Pitta-Kapha constitution, typical of many competitive athletes. Larry is primarily a Vata. Working out like his father would be exhausting for his less rugged constitution.

Here are some general exercise guidelines for the three main body types, Vata, Pitta, and Kapha. Remember, almost everyone is a combination of two or occasionally all three body types, usually with one predominating. Refer to the results of the Body Type Quiz you took in Chapter 2, or to what you learned from consulting an Ayurvedic physician.

Vata types are generally light, limber, and quick. They do not have the physique for contact sports, and since their physical energy comes in bursts, they often lack the stamina for rugged continuous exercise such as long-distance running, rowing, or competitive swimming. Light aerobic exercise is best, along with any activity that emphasizes balance and flexibility. Speedy, restless Vatas may be attracted to high-action sports like racquetball, but what they need is just the opposite: something that will help them settle down. Yoga is a good choice, as are golf and walking.

If you have a Vata constitution, you need to be careful not to overdo physical activity. Respect your body's capacity and don't overexert. Vatas are impulsive and tend to push themselves past the point of fatigue toward exhaustion. Be especially attentive to your body's signals; "listen" to what your body is saying and don't push past the "breaking point," where you begin to sweat and breathe heavily.

This is especially important for the elderly. According to Ayurveda, *Vata increases in everyone's makeup in later life.* For safety, it is vital not to strain.

Physical exhaustion throws anyone's Vata out of balance. If you feel "wiped out" by exercise, if you experience insomnia or joint pain, or if you feel more anxious or restless when you increase your exercise level, these are all signs that Vata is aggravated and your exercise may be doing you more harm than good. Cut back on the type, amount, or intensity of exercise. Perhaps you should be doing only some slow-paced jogging or brisk walking, which will have a calming effect on Vata if done in moderation.

Also, since Vata is considered to be cold and dry in nature, Vata body types should avoid exercising outdoors in winter or breathing cold, dry air. Both of these can aggravate Vata and lead to respiratory difficulties.

Ann is a thin, energetic 26-year-old jazz and ballet dancer who, due to her profession, is highly motivated to remain thin. In addition to dieting, she uses vigorous exercise as a means to this end. She runs approximately five miles a day, six days per week. But over the last year, she gradually developed insomnia, fatigue, and occasional bouts of anxiety.

After taking a course in Ayurveda at a community center, Ann realized that she was exercising in a manner that was incompatible with her body type. With a primarily Vata constitution, she needed to push herself much less. She slowed the pace and frequency of her jogging, "listened" better to her body in order to avoid overexercise, incorporated the Sun Salutation in her regimen, and ate a more nourishing, balanced diet. With these few adjustments, over a few months Ann's symptoms faded away and she felt stronger and had more energy and endurance for her dancing.

Pitta types are medium in build and tend to have medium strength and endurance. Because Pittas are by nature driven to succeed, they bring determination to their exercise. They like competitive sports—so long as they win. Physical activity that lacks challenge is usually too boring, which makes walking seem unattractive at first. And yet no one benefits more from a good walk than does a Pitta personality. This is because Pittas, often intoxicated by work, deadlines, and pressure, need to take time out every day to relax, breathe fresh air, and be in a beautiful natural setting.

Because Pitta imbalance may be correlated with increased irritability and anger, Pittas should think twice about getting into ferociously competitive tennis, squash, handball, or even golf matches. Pittas are strong enough on will power and drive, but weak on relaxation. They have a hard time just enjoying themselves, but this is just what will help them remain in balance.

Being hot by nature, the Pitta constitution is a good candidate for swimming. Many Pitta businesspeople find that a visit to the pool is excellent for relieving tension and toning the whole system. But don't drive yourself to do a set number of laps every time. Keep the activity mild and enjoyable. And be extra careful not to overdo in hot weather. When engaging in competitive sports, learn to focus on enjoying the process rather than on being completely goal oriented. Remind yourself that having fun and getting good exercise is more important than winning.

Ralph, a 52-year-old red-headed car salesman with a medium build, was notorious on the golf course for throwing down his club and cursing whenever he made a poor shot. Although he claimed he "loved this game," he began to develop an ulcer that seemed to get aggravated whenever he went out on the golf course. Antacids helped, but he took his wife's advice and visited a doctor who integrated Ayurvedic approaches into his medical practice.

The doctor made only a few recommendations: daily meditation, a Pitta-pacifying diet, some cooling herbs, and doing a brief coconut oil self-massage prior to his golf matches. He also suggested that Ralph swing his club with only three quarters of his usual force, and that for a few weeks he play without a scorecard and spend more time enjoying the scenery.

Taking his attention away from the competitive aspect, along with the Ayurvedic recommendations, dramatically reduced Ralph's Pitta imbalance. Forgetting about the score and "enjoying the process" not only helped heal the ulcer, but actually improved his score when he began carrying the scorecard again. Less driven and more relaxed, he found his game spontaneously improving.

Kapha types are the strongest of the three Ayurvedic body types and have exceptional endurance. Solid and heavyset, Kaphas often turn out to be natural baseball and football players, particularly if a good proportion of Pitta is present in their makeup to add drive and competitiveness. (If Vata is added, however, the excellent endurance and muscle strength can be considerably reduced.)

Kaphas benefit more from hard, sustained exercise than does anyone else. It makes them feel invigorated to work up a good sweat. This is because excess Kapha that has built up as toxins in the body is expelled during a hard workout.

Kaphas are natural candidates for becoming "couch potatoes." They tend toward a sedentary lifestyle and often need a lot of motivation to get them going. If your constitution is largely Kapha, don't wait for a heart attack or a high cholesterol count to motivate you with fear. To maintain balance, take up running, jogging, aerobics, rowing, or some other vigorous exercise early in life and sustain it. This will pay off right now: You will feel much more vital and alive. It will also probably do good things for your cholesterol, which may tend to be high, for your overweight, and for any other signs of physical inertia.

This recommendation that Kaphas engage in more vigorous activity should not be seen as a contradiction to the general advice not to strain. Kapha types, endowed with greater physical strength and endurance, can usually do a lot more vigorous exercise before they begin to reach their "breaking point" and feel strained. (This will obviously not be true if you are overweight and out of shape, when great caution is needed in beginning an exercise program. If you fit this description, it's best to consult your doctor before embarking on any exercise program.)

Like Vatas, Kaphas should be careful not to exercise outdoors in winter. A warm gym is a good place to get your exercise during those cold months. Having a vigorous warm sesame oil massage will also help to move any excess Kapha out of the system.

Mary, a 40-year-old physician with dark, wavy hair and a strong, sturdy stature complained of having low energy and occasional depression, especially in the winter and early spring seasons. She tried anti-depressants, but found them of only marginal benefit. As she was a little overweight, she wanted to go on a diet but the stress of work made dieting difficult because she found food "a relaxant."

As a result of taking an introductory course in Maharishi Ayurveda for physicians, Mary learned that she had a Kapha imbalance and decided to prescribe several Kapha-pacifying measures for herself. The dietary changes and herbs were helpful, but she found that she got the most benefit from joining a health club. Starting from her condition of low energy, she gradually built up her endurance to the point where she could play 30 minutes of racquetball about four times a week. To her surprise, she not only lost weight but also began to feel lighter and more energetic. Her depression gradually gave way to a consistent happy and bouyant mood.

Do It Daily: 10 Tips for Working Exercise Into Your Day

Most of us have decided to exercise more, made New Year's resolutions, joined health clubs, bought exercise equipment . . . but despite our best intentions, other commitments and time constraints usually interfere. The following suggestions will help you integrate exercise into your daily and weekly routine.

- Walk to work, or at least part of the way.
- Take a walk when you get home, or after dinner. Go with your spouse or a friend. In the words of Dean Ornish, M.D., author of the best-selling book, *Dr. Dean Ornish's Program for Reversing Heart Disease*, "Talk about your day; use the time to unwind and build friendship and intimacy."
- Schedule your walks or exercise sessions. Write them into your calendar as fixed appointments. Appointments with yourself

CHOOSE A SPORT FOR YOUR BODY TYPE

The following charts will help you select the sports and exercises most suitable to your body type. Please note that these lists are not exhaustive, but are just suggestions.

Vata: Vata types will naturally excel at fast-paced sports requiring speed, agility, and quick bursts of energy. However, sports that will have a balancing effect on Vata are slow and calming, such as

yoga	bowling
swimming	sailing
volleyball	weight training
horseback riding	golf
easy bicycle touring	canoeing and easy rowing
hiking and walking	nonviolent martial arts such as Tai Chi
archery	baseball/softball

If you engage in vigorous sports, be sure not to overexert. Take plenty of breaks if you're noticing any of the warning signs such as pounding heart, profuse sweating, need to breathe through your mouth, etc.

Pitta: Persons with Pitta constitutions will be drawn toward sports that call upon their natural athletic strength, speed, and stamina. However, some sports will help to balance the highly competitive spirit—as well as the physiology—of Pitta types and will offer the possibility of pure enjoyment rather than competition. These include

downhill skiing	cycling
kayaking/rowing	wind surfing
sailing	surfing
mountain biking	martial arts
golf	water skiing
touch football	basketball and other team sports
diving	horseback riding
recreational cross-country skiing	noncompetitive swimming
ice skating	
yoga	

Kapha: Kapha types excel in endurance and strength. Because of their warm, affable nature they like team sports. But sports to help Kapha types maintain balance must be stimulating and vigorous. Such sports include

aerobics	body building
basketball	cycling
calisthenics	racquetball

(Box text continues on page 118)

fencing
lacrosse
javelin
sculling
martial arts
gymnastics
tennis
stair stepping
roller blading
cross-country running

handball
volleyball
shot put
swimming
soccer
rock climbing
rowing
parcourse running
cross-country skiing

The above charts are adapted from Chapter 8, "Sports by Body Type," in *Body, Mind and Sport* by John Douillard (Harmony Books, 1994).

---

for your health and longevity are certainly as important as any business engagement. A few minutes of Sun Salutations and Yoga postures as a regular part of your Ayurvedic morning routine (see Chapter 6) is an ideal way to ensure some quality exercise every day.

- Ride a bike. Millions of people in Europe and Asia ride a bicycle to work or to do minor shopping. This idea is catching on in many U. S. cities, where special bicycle lanes are being set aside.

- Use the stairs instead of the elevator.

- Go dancing. Ballroom dancing or the latest rock moves aren't the only alternatives. Try line dancing, folk dancing, square dancing.

- Start any exercise program slowly. If you push too hard at the beginning and burn out, you will understandably lose the motivation to continue. Do a little, regularly, and gradually increase your time and exertion level.

- For many people, the only way to exercise regularly is to make a commitment to a class (aerobics, dance, tennis, yoga, whatever). If you pay for it and tell people you are doing it, your chances are better.

- Make commitments to other people. Have them come to pick you up or promise to pick them up or to meet them at set times and places.

- Most important: Choose activities you enjoy. The key to success in anything in life is sticking with it regularly over an extended period of time. You can't become a good writer, doctor, baseball player, engineer, or even a good parent or spouse unless you keep at it. The same is true for deriving maximum benefit from an exercise program.

  Discipline and determination, with an eye toward the future, may get you through medical school, but it probably won't keep you exercising. You have to enjoy what you do. So create an exercise plan that is fun for you. If you are a person who loves quiet walks in the open air, the best exercise for you is not likely to be an indoor aerobics class accompanied by loud rock music.

Exercise has both short- and long-term benefits for your health, your productivity, and your feeling of vitality. If you are one of the 85 percent of Americans who don't exercise regularly, I hope the information in this chapter will encourage you to do something that will pay high dividends for years to come.

A Word of Caution

No matter how healthy you may be, I strongly recommend that you structure your exercise program with your doctor's participation, especially if you are over 40. Certainly if you have a cardiac condition or any serious health condition you need to be guided by a physician in developing an exercise program.

Discuss this book and the principles in it with your doctor, or with a physician trained in Ayurveda. Work with him or her in developing your "exercise prescription." Most doctors will readily see the value of minimizing your risk by keeping your exercise level to 50 percent of capacity. Again, exercising to more than 50 percent of capacity is not advisable for anyone other than a competitive athlete.

It is also very important for you to know when to stop exercising. Here are six danger signs:

- Panting or shortness of breath
- Unusually heavy perspiration
- Undue fatigue
- Dizziness

- Heartbeat faster than your target range
- Pain in your chest, back, or arms that does not go away when you slow down your pace

See your doctor *without delay* if you experience any of the above danger signals during or after your exercise session.

CHAPTER 8

REVITALIZING AND HEALING WITH HERBS

Today in the era of modern medicine we tend to think that medicines are invented in the high-tech laboratories of giant pharmaceutical companies by research chemists wearing white coats. But for thousands of years, herbal medicines derived from local plants have been the primary means of healing in all parts of the world and continue to be widely used.

These days we often see pictures on our TV screens of tribal medicine men climbing trees and poking through dense rain-forest undergrowth in search of medicinal leaves and roots, as Western scientists trail behind, taking notes and gathering samples to bring back to the laboratory. But it's not just obscure forest tribes who use herbs; herbal remedies are used worldwide and remain at the core of the ancient, sophisticated medical systems used by hundreds of millions of people in China and India.

Many modern medicines are derived from plants, some of them used for centuries in natural healing. Reserpine, a drug formerly employed to control schizophrenia and now used to treat high blood pressure, is derived from the root of the plant *rauwolfia serpentina*. Digitalis, famous for its ability to combat heart failure and heart irregularities, originally came from the plant *digitalis purpurea*. Many antibiotics are derived from chemicals naturally secreted from fungi; penicillin, first discovered as a mold on bread, is a prime example.

In addition, many common herbs used in kitchens the world over can be used for healing and for balancing our minds and bodies. As you will learn in this chapter, these include ginger, turmeric, cinnamon, cloves, coriander, garlic, black pepper, and many more.

According to experts, Ayurveda probably has "the oldest, most visionary, most developed science of herbal medicine in the world." Ayurvedic physicians have described and classified (according to their effects and benefits) literally thousands of herbs and herbal compounds, subjecting them to the test of everyday use for more than 3,000 years.

In this chapter you will learn how and why these herbs work and how you can put them to use easily and inexpensively for prevention, healing, purification, and rejuvenation.

Herbs—Nature's Own Medicines

In simplest terms, herbs are plants. They may be large plants, such as trees, or tiny plants almost impossible to find. Either the entire plant, or some part of it—root, leaf, stem, bark, flower, or seed— may be useful for medicinal purposes.

We can also look at herbs as foods, highly concentrated in certain beneficial nutrients. They may be useful for the health of a particular part of the body (such as the liver, stomach, or other organs, the tissues, nervous system, etc.) or for the body as a whole. These latter herbs, known as *rasayanas* or rejuvenators, build immunity, well-being, and vitality for the entire system.

Some herbs have a cleansing effect, for example, on the stomach, lungs, blood, or colon. Others are used to treat imbalance or to maintain and promote balance in the doshas, those qualities of Vata, Pitta, and Kapha that underlie our body's constitutional type.

The easiest and most common ways of using herbs are (1) to mix the chopped, powdered, or whole fresh herbs in with your food, (2) take them powdered in capsules, or (3) boil them in water to make a tea. Other ways herbs can be taken are heated in milk, cooked into a medicinal ghee, or eaten with a little honey.

Why Don't We Use Herbs More?

Herbs are entirely natural, inexpensive (except for some rare varieties), and, perhaps most wonderful, aren't likely to generate the kinds of side effects that may result from many modern medicines. So why have we gotten away from using them, turning instead to synthetic drugs?

Probably the main reason is purely economic. The enormous multinational drug companies make billions of dollars mass manufacturing medicines for worldwide distribution. These drugs are heavily promoted to doctors in medical journals and to the public in the mass media, where we cannot escape being told every day of the wonders of the latest pain reliever, cold remedy, or heartburn formula.

These powerful modern drugs are almost miraculous at relieving symptoms. This is because modern chemistry can extract or synthesize what is called the "active ingredient" in an herb, the chemical that appears to produce the desired effect of relieving a certain symptom. In our fast-paced world, we look for the quick fix. We have no time for a recuperation period; we need to get right back to work, to our numerous responsibilities.

But these modern drugs often have serious side effects, partly because of this process of extracting the "active ingredient," separating it from the wholeness of the plant. Antibiotics, for example, frequently cause yeast infections and abdominal problems such as diarrhea. Worse, bacteria develop resistance to the antibiotics, so increasingly powerful drugs are needed to kill infections, and the strains of bacteria that survive become more and more deadly.

Medicines for high blood pressure frequently cause depression and fatigue. Steroids can result in ulcers and osteoporosis. In fact, virtually all modern medicines carry some risks, some of them quite severe. Just recently, studies have revealed that estrogen, routinely prescribed to millions of menopausal women, seems to significantly increase a woman's chances of developing breast cancer.

No wonder, then, that so many people are turning back toward natural herbal medicine. And they are turning back with a passion. A recent study in a major medical journal surprised health care professionals by reporting that Americans actually paid more out-of-pocket money for alternative medical approaches than for standard Western treatments.

When correctly prescribed, herbs are devoid of side effects and often have *side benefits*. Ginger, for example, may be taken as a stimulant for the appetite and digestion, but in addition to improving digestion it helps in the reduction of fatigue, is healing to colds and coughs, and helps eliminate abdominal gas.

Herbs have a special place in the growing wellness movement in our society, a movement that reflects our desire to take more control over our own health care and live a long, healthy life. Many people are dissatisfied with the modern system of medicine. Rather than *disease treatment,* people want proactive *health care.*

Herbs are a central part of the solution. Along with a diet and exercise plan tailored to your body type and a daily routine more in tune with natural rhythms, you can use herbs to help prevent illness, balance your mind and body, enhance your immune system, and promote a more positive state of overall health and well-being.

Putting Herbs to Work for You

A fundamental principle of Ayurveda is the interconnectedness of everything in nature. Thousands of years ago the Vedic sages of India clearly realized what only the leading-edge thinkers of today, in physics, ecology, and other sciences, have realized: that life is an interrelated, interdependent whole.

Nature, from solid surface structures to subtle subatomic energy fields, is the same everywhere. Everything is made up of the same fundamental materials and is organized by the same intelligence, the same laws of nature. This law of uniformity or complementarity holds, as Deepak Chopra, M.D., expresses it, that "nature thinks everywhere alike." That means that despite surface differences, plants, minerals, and human bodies, as well as every other item of nature, are closely related on the deeper, *quantum* levels.

On the quantum level, all matter is made up of energy. This energy is not static, but moves in waves. A basic Ayurvedic principle is that the wave frequencies of certain plants perfectly match the wave frequencies of various parts of the body.

Disease occurs when something in the body gets "out of phase" or "out of synch"; its wave pattern becomes distorted, often by some form of stress.

This is where the healing power of herbs comes in. An herb can resonate with its "match" in the body, to realign the deeper wavelike nature of the organ or tissue and to reestablish normal and healthy functioning. In Dr. Chopra's words:

> The liver, for example, is built up from a specific sequence of vibrations at the quantum level. In the case of liver malfunction, some dis-

ruption of the proper sequence in these vibrations is at fault. According to Ayurveda, an herb exists with this exact same sequence, and when applied, it restores the liver's functioning.

It has been the genius of the Ayurvedic physicians—and other experts in herbs around the world—to discover which herbs produce which effects. In Ayurveda, this classification is vast and sophisticated. What follows in the next section is just a tiny introduction to it. You won't really need to know all this when you use herbs, but you might feel comforted that such a deep science underlies the Ayurvedic herbal recommendations, a science that thoroughly understands and can predict the effects of these gifts of nature on our mind-body system, based on centuries of application.

Harness the Healing Power of Herbs

Ayurvedic herbs are classified according to dozens of factors, such as taste, "action," effect on digestive fire (*agni*), post-digestive effect, energy, attribute, special potency, and many more. Let's look at a few important ones:

Taste

Like each food, every herb has a specific taste. When the tongue picks up the taste, the entire physiology is affected, as are the three doshas, Vata, Pitta, and Kapha. Bitter herbs such as turmeric generally reduce Pitta and Kapha. They help to curtail rashes and infections (inflammations largely due to Pitta) and to reduce mucus (a sign of aggravated Kapha). On the opposite side, sweet herbs such as licorice generally increase Kapha and reduce Pitta and Vata.

Here is a summary of the effects of the six tastes:

Taste	*Vata*	*Pitta*	*Kapha*
Salt	↓	↑	↑
Sweet	↓	↓	↑
Sour	↓	↑	↑
Bitter	↑	↓	↓
Pungent	↑	↑	↓
Astringent	↑	↓	↓

Health tip: The added flavor that herbs give to our food is important beyond the realm of mere enjoyment. Before we swallow a mouthful of food, long before it hits the stomach and begins to be broken down and assimilated, the smell and taste stimulate digestive juices in the stomach, pancreas, and gall bladder. These juices prepare the body to receive the food.

If our food is excessively bland (or stale, left over, canned, frozen, processed, etc., with little lively taste), it will not stimulate the *agni* or digestive juices properly and is likely to be incompletely digested. This produces *ama*, inadequately digested food that isn't fully metabolized, from the Ayurvedic perspective the first step in the process of disease formation.

Qualities

Of the 20 key qualities Ayurveda recognizes throughout nature, six are most important when it comes to herbs and food: hot/cold, wet/dry, heavy/light. Vata is dry, cold, and light. Pitta is light, hot, and slightly moist. Kapha is heavy, wet, and cold. In considering which herbs to use, the key principle is that opposite qualities balance the disorder. So an herb that is hot in property, such as *pippali* (Indian long pepper) or ginger, is balancing to disorders of Vata and Kapha, while an herb that is cold and heavy (such as aloe) is balancing to Pitta.

Potency

Like the yin/yang dichotomy in Chinese natural medicine, potency refers to the two main types of energy the body will acquire from any food or herb. These are classified as heating and cooling.

Herbs that are cooling mostly have sweet, astringent, and bitter tastes. They pacify Pitta and tend to increase Kapha and Vata. These are helpful for reducing inflammation and other conditions associated with too much heat in the system, such as liver, skin, and stomach disorders. A typical cooling herb is golden seal, which is bitter in taste and helpful in cooling the body and reducing fever.

Heating herbs and foods are pungent, sour, and salty. They increase Pitta and pacify or reduce Vata and Kapha. They are helpful in conditions in which digestion and metabolism are weak and need stimulation. A simple example is warm water with lemon juice, which improves digestion and reduces ama.

Other Factors

Herbs also have what is called a post-digestive effect, also known as the aftertaste or *vipaka* in Sanskrit. This refers to the effect the food or herb will have after it has been digested, which is sometimes different from the immediate effect of the taste. Ginger has a pungent taste but a sweet aftertaste or post-digestive effect.

Another important property of herbs is its special potency (*prabhava*). This refers to a special effect an herb sometimes has that could not be predicted from its taste or other qualities. Basil, for example, has heating properties, yet brings down fever.

The therapeutic effect of each herb results from a combination of all of the above factors.

Now that we have looked at what makes these herbs work, let's move on to some practical advice about how to use them.

Herbs You Can Use to Stimulate Appetite and Digestion

Improving the efficiency of your digestive system is no small matter, as Ayurveda holds that inadequate digestion is at the root of virtually all illness (see Chapter 10).

The easiest way to stimulate appetite and digestion is with pungent herbs. I have already mentioned the use of a "ginger pickle"—about half a teaspoon of raw grated ginger mixed with lemon juice and a pinch of salt—taken before meals to get the digestive juices flowing. Other pungent herbs that can be used in cooking to improve appetite (even their smell will help as the food is cooking) include basil, bay leaves, black pepper, cardamom, cayenne, cinnamon, cloves, coriander, cumin, garlic, ginger, horseradish, mustard seeds, oregano, peppermint, sage, and thyme.

Salt is technically not an herb, but can be used in small doses, especially by Vata body types, to promote salivation and increase appetite and digestive power. Both Pittas and Kaphas need to moderate salt intake, since too much salt can be aggravating to both.

Chewing on a clove or on some cardamom seeds occasionally during the day will aid digestion.

If you have too much Pitta in your system, as evidenced perhaps by chronic heartburn or even ulcers, two teaspoons of fresh aloe vera gel two or three times a day should improve digestion without increasing acidity.

Don't forget that one of the easiest and best ways to increase your appetite and improve your digestion is to eat in tune with nature's daily cycles of Vata, Pitta, and Kapha. High noon is the peak of Pitta time, and it is then that our digestive fires are naturally highest. People with Pitta body types are generally ravenously hungry by noon and should feed that fire on time. The rest of us will find our appetites stronger and our digestive process more effective if we get in the habit of eating our biggest meal for lunch. See Chapter 6 for a more complete discussion.

Herbs for Cleansing and Purification

Ayurveda considers reduction of ama (accumulated wastes, toxins, and incompletly digested food) as the first step in treating virtually all health problems. If the system is clogged with impurities, herbs cannot be very effective. All the pungent herbs mentioned earlier are helpful for cleansing the system of these accumulated wastes, as stimulation of agni naturally dissolves ama.

As we've seen, ama has characteristics similar to Kapha—it is heavy, sticky, and cold. Pungent herbs, with their natural heating properties, kindle the body's digestive fires, which then automatically begin to burn off the accumulated ama. The easy-to-find pungent herbs are mentioned under "Herbs to Stimulate Appetite and Digestion."

Bitter herbs also combat ama by preventing it from building up. Although they are cooling in nature and not stimulating to agni, their natural effect is to detoxify. They are antibacterial and anti-inflammatory and are cleansing to the blood and tissues. Common bitter herbs include aloe, chrysanthemum, dandelion, echinacea, gentian, golden seal, rhubarb, and yellow dock.

Another, more involved cleansing and purification procedure that you can't do at home but that you should know about is called *panchakarma.* (This is a Sanskrit word that means "five actions.") Panchakarma is a series of treatments offered at various Ayurvedic clinics. The purpose is to dislodge and flush out built-up ama or impurities from the body and restore balance to your mind-body system. The steps of purification include a laxative to flush out the intestinal tract, oil massage to loosen the impurities, sweat treatments, medicated enemas, and several others.

Herbs, both to treat imbalances and to promote vitality and longevity, work best after panchakarma, which is recommended at regular (approximately four-month) intervals throughout the year. See Appendix B for a partial listing of places you can receive panchakarma treatments.

Other ways to help cleanse the system of ama include eating a lighter, preferably vegetarian diet, with less fat and sugar; light fasting by skipping one or two meals per week; and sipping hot water at intervals of half an hour to an hour during the day. Exercise, by increasing agni, helps to eliminate ama. Also the increased body heat and sweating have a purifying effect by enhancing elimination of body impurities.

Use These Herbs to Heal and Create Balance

Most health problems are understood in Ayurveda as being caused by an imbalance in Vata, Pitta, or Kapha. Specific herbs can be used to reduce the accumulation of the doshas, thus helping to restore balance and heal the problem.

Vata imbalances often relate to the brain, mind, and nervous system. Common disorders include insomnia, anxiety, and pain conditions such as arthritis. Muscle tension, signs and symptoms of advanced aging, and problems with any function of movement in the body such as respiration, elimination, and circulation are likely to be related to excess Vata.

Vata-balancing herbs include anise, asafoetida, cinnamon, cumin, ginger, gotu kola (helps calm the mind), licorice, natural sugar, nutmeg, rock salt, sesame seeds, and valerian (helps sleep). Castor oil and a tea made from castor root are considered highly beneficial for pacifying and balancing Vata. For example, a common Vata imbalance is arthritis. A helpful prescription for arthritis is one teaspoon of castor oil in ginger tea at bedtime. Use less oil if this amount is too stimulating to your elimination process.

Pitta imbalances manifest largely as problems with the digestive system, such as ulcers, diarrhea, and colitis. Thyroid and other hormonal disorders frequently have their origin in aggravated Pitta. Eye problems, infections, and inflammation, as well as most skin disorders, are due to too much heat (Pitta) in the system.

Pitta-balancing herbs to reduce aggravated Pitta include aloe, burdock, chrysanthemum, coconut, coriander, cumin, fennel, golden seal, mint, pomegranate, sandalwood, *shatavari* (Indian asparagus), natural sugar, and turmeric.

Although ginger is pungent and heating, its post-digestive effect is sweet; if used in moderation it can also help balance Pitta.

Kapha imbalances are due to an accumulation of too much tissue or fluid in the system. Typical Kapha disorders include colds, coughs, bronchitis and other lung problems, sinus congestion, swelling, obesity, and tumors.

Kapha-balancing herbs are generally warming and drying. They include alfalfa, basil, black pepper, cardamom, cinnamon, cloves, cumin, eucalyptus, fenugreek, garlic, ginger, Indian long pepper (*pippali*), peppermint, sarsaparilla, spearmint, turmeric, and wintergreen.

Herbs for Rejuvenation and Revitalization

The herbs we will talk about now form one of the most wonderful aspects of Ayurveda: the promotion of perfect health and longevity. Ayurvedic medicine is concerned with far more than the treatment of imbalances and full-grown illnesses; its emphasis is on prevention of disease, promotion of health, and enhancement of the quality of life.

To help us accomplish this positive state of wellness, Ayurveda has developed a wealth of herbs and herbal compounds. These are called *rasayanas,* which means enlivening *rasa* (plasma), according to Ayurveda the first product of digestion that nourishes every aspect of the mind and body. Rasa is like the sap in a tree; it provides the basic nutrition out of which the whole structure of the tree is formed.

The expression, "Well begun is half done" explains the importance of rasa. On page 73 we saw the chain of events leading to the formation of all the body's tissues, beginning with rasa and leading up to the creation of ojas. If rasa is of excellent quality and free of impurities, there is a strong likelihood the rest of the tissues will form properly and be of similarly excellent, healthy quality.

Herbs that are considered to have a vitalizing, rejuvenating effect include *ashvagandha* (winter cherry), *bala* (Indian country mallow), *shatavari* (asparagus root), *amalaki,* and *brahmi* (gotu kola).

Garlic is also very strengthening, but tends to produce some dullness of mind. Both garlic and onions can stimulate sexual energy and are not recommended for those pursuing a spiritual path involving celibacy.

The compound *chyavanprash*, a sweet herbal jelly comprising numerous herbs, is used throughout India for rejuvenation and strengthening. Various brands are available in this country at Indian groceries and natural food stores. Another product similarly available is *Maharishi Amrit Kalash*, an ancient blend of herbs, fruits, honey, and ghee, that has been shown to increase endorphins and enhance immunity.

Nonherbal foods considered especially strengthening to both mind and body are almonds, dates, honey, milk, raisins, sesame seeds, and ghee. In practical Ayurvedic usage, many herbs are taken with milk, honey, or ghee.

Other rejuvenative and tonic herbs are fo-ti, ginseng, and wild yam.

Herbs for Common Health Concerns

Important: Always consult a physician if a problem persists or is more severe, perhaps requiring a combined (Western and Ayurvedic) approach.

Abdominal gas: Add 1/2 teaspoon each of ginger and cardamom, with a pinch of asafoetida, to 2 cups of water. Boil until only 1/2 to 1 cup remains and drink as a tea. In addition you can chew fennel seeds after meals or at various times during the day.

Burns: Apply ghee directly to the affected area. This can produce amazingly effective results. Alternatively, use aloe vera gel. Coconut oil is also effective. With ghee or coconut oil, a little turmeric can be added.

Colds: Use ginger and turmeric in cooking. Drink ginger tea. Take the herb echinacea either as a tea or as a tincture. Add some honey to the tea, but only after the tea cools to sipping temperature. Eat a light diet, consisting mostly of warm teas and soups. Avoid dairy, cold foods, sweets, and fried foods.

Constipation: Take two teaspoons of psyllium husk powder in warm water at bedtime. Or take a cup of warm milk with a teaspoon or two of ghee once or twice a day.

Diarrhea: Mix 1/4 to 1/2 cup yogurt with an equal amount of water, add 1/4 teaspoon each of ginger, nutmeg, and cumin powder. Drink several times a day.

Earache: Heat a clove of garlic in hot sesame oil for about 5 minutes. Let stand until the oil is only slightly warm. (Test the oil temperature on the back of your hand to be sure it's not too hot.) Then apply 2 or 3 drops in the affected ear.

Irritated eyes: Apply a few drops of sterile rose water in each eye several times a day until the condition clears. Or make a very mild, dilute solution of turmeric water by boiling 1/4 teaspoon turmeric in 1 glass of water; strain; let cool. Then apply 2 to 3 drops several times per day (with a sterile dropper) in the affected eye. Make a fresh batch each day. To keep pure during the day, cover with Saran Wrap.

Low back pain: Make a paste of ginger powder and apply to the lower back for 15 to 30 minutes. Also, massage with sesame or almond oil followed by a hot bath or hot tub or hot-water bottle.

Sinus headache: Drink ginger tea. Make a paste of ginger powder mixed with water and apply warm to forehead. Avoid fried foods, sweets, dairy, cold foods and drinks.

Sore throat: Gargle with warm turmeric water or salt water. Or suck on cardamom seeds throughout the day.

Skin problems (especially acne): Twice a day apply a paste of turmeric or sandalwood powder mixed with water (or you can combine the two powders). Often tumeric cream is available at health food stores; it works great. Or apply aloe vera gel instead. Use more turmeric as seasoning in your food. Drink aloe vera juice, one tablespoon two or three times a day.

Herbs are nature's gift to us. The ancient Ayurvedic tradition has used them effectively for thousands of years. If you've never used herbs before for healing, try getting your feet wet with some common household herbs, such as ginger or turmeric, for some of the purposes described here. I'm sure you will be pleased with the results.

PART 3

AYURVEDIC STRATEGIES FOR COMMON HEALTH PROBLEMS

NATURAL CURE FOR COLDS, COUGHS, AND SINUS PROBLEMS

Jennifer's colds were about as predictable as the seasons. From the time she was a little girl she seemed to have a cold every winter that dragged on for weeks or even months. Then in the spring, she had another one. She consumed a lot of over-the-counter cold remedies to help stop her runny noses, but the side effects—dry mouth, dry eyes, pounding heart, sleepiness—began to be almost as uncomfortable as the cold symptoms. For awhile she just gave up and assumed it was her fate—until, when she was in her mid-forties, a friend suggested she look into Ayurveda.

Very interested in finding a natural way to combat her colds without unpleasant side effects, she consulted an Ayurvedic physician who helped her understand the underlying causes of her seemingly endless battle with colds.

The first thing she found out was that she had a predominantly Vata body type, but that rather than being in balance so she could enjoy the positive qualities of Vata, her lifestyle exaggerated and unbalanced her Vata and her health reflected it. Probably the worst offender was her schedule; she often stayed up late and tended to get along on less sleep than she needed, so she was always pushing herself a little and was always a little tired.

135

Also typical of Vatas, her eating habits were quite unpredictable. Mealtimes depended on whether or not she was hungry and what she might be doing at the time; she rarely took time to cook much in the way of fresh foods. With a light build (she had been an aspiring dancer in her teens and twenties), she could get away with eating pretty much anything she wanted—or so she thought—because she didn't gain weight if she ate lots of pizza and pasta, cheese sandwiches, creamy desserts, and so on. She also ran several miles four or five times a week, which helped keep her figure trim.

What happened to her, however, is that her escalating sleep debt, plus what was really too much exercise for her body type, weakened her immune system and made her susceptible to cold viruses. At the same time her diet, heavy in Kapha-producing foods, clogged up her system with mucus that began discharging liberally as soon as a cold began.

With a few lifestyle changes suggested by the Ayurvedic doctor—a more regular schedule, a more balancing diet, and a few specific suggestions for herbal teas and appropriate exercise—Jennifer was able to get the upper hand and gain a freedom from colds she never thought possible.

But rather than go into the specific treatments prescribed for Jennifer, in the rest of this chapter I'll tell you what *you* can do to prevent and treat colds. First, though, I'd like to take a minute to explain what colds are and point out the inadequacies in our current ways of treating them.

Why We Get Colds

From an Ayurvedic perspective, there are several key factors in catching a cold. They are:

1. Decreased immunity
2. Dry or irritated sinuses and mucous membranes
3. Excess Kapha in the system due to improper diet
4. Ama (impurity) in the body due to poor digestion

Let's look at these briefly.

Decreased Immunity.   Fatigue, depression, lack of exercise, poor nutrition, or other factors depress the immune system and permit the growth of viruses in the respiratory system. As everyone knows, our bodies are subjected to a bombardment of billions of germs every day, yet we usually remain healthy. When the effectiveness of our immune system becomes sub-par, those bacteria and viruses have a chance to develop.

Dry or Irritated Mucous Membranes.   Our mucous membranes may become dry for many reasons, such as living in an arid climate; some unusually dry, windy weather; or the effects of home heating in wintry weather. Or they might become irritated and inflamed, as in the case of allergies, where pollen in the air irritates the delicate membranes and causes swelling. Both the dryness (a Vata condition), and the inflammation (a condition of aggravated Pitta) weaken the respiratory tissue and make it more susceptible to viruses.

Excess Kapha.   Diet, in particular a Kapha-increasing diet, is usually a major contributing factor in developing a cold. This is especially true when any of the other factors (decreased immunity, dryness, or inflammation) are also present. When a person eats too much Kapha-producing food (such as cold food; fried food; milk; cheese; eggs; yogurt; ice cream; desserts made of flour, sugar, and shortening; fatty meats) the excess Kapha from these foods tends to produce mucus.

The mucus is manufactured primarily in the stomach, one of the principle seats of Kapha. When Kapha builds up in the stomach, it tends to spread through the lymphatic and circulatory systems to the respiratory systems, where it may accumulate further.

Our bodies attempt to eliminate this excess Kapha by way of the mucous membranes in the upper respiratory tract. Thus, the sinus and nasal passages become the highway through which the excess mucus is removed. Clearing out this accumulated gunk is a good thing—mucus serves as a culture medium for bacterial infection—but the process is likely to take the form of sinus congestion and/or a cold.

Ama in the Body.   Overeating, and eating too quickly, both result in the formation of ama. Ama is food that has not been properly digested and assimilated, which then becomes unusable to the body.

Ama eventually becomes toxic and is a key factor in disease formation. Excess mucus is a form of ama.

Cold Medicines Are Only Partially Effective

The standard approach to treating colds these days is to attack the symptoms. The available medications, whether over the counter or prescribed, aim primarily at drying up the swollen and inflamed mucous membranes. Although these medications can be effective in reducing cold symptoms while the drug is acting, they have several drawbacks.

- They don't actually treat any of the underlying causes of the cold—decreased immunity, ama in the system, etc.
- The side effects—such as dry mouth and eyes, and especially drowsiness—are often as bad as the cold symptoms themselves and can even be dangerous. Sleepiness while driving or working with machinery could result in injury or even death.

So while it may be helpful to use these medicines in the short run, they fall far short of the ideal. Ideally, treatment for colds would be natural and free of side effects; it would address the actual causes of the cold and help prevent future occurrences by building immunity and improving the diet and digestion. These form the basis of the Ayurvedic approach.

Use Food to Prevent and Cure Colds

The main reason we accumulate excess mucus is that our diet contains too much Kapha-increasing food. A balanced diet will go a long way toward maintaining good health without colds and sinus problems, while an imbalanced diet is the shortcut to illness.

Here, a balanced diet means eating all six tastes (see Chapter 3) in proper proportion. To refresh your memory, here is a rundown of the six tastes:

1. **Sweet** (including milk, grains, anything with sugar or honey)
2. **Salt** (any salty food)
3. **Sour** (cheese, yogurt, vinegar, citrus fruits)
4. **Bitter** (green leafy vegetables)
5. **Pungent** (spicy or peppery foods, horseradish, onions, garlic)
6. **Astringent** (beans and lentils, pomegranates, cabbage)

A cold can easily develop when we take in too many foods with sweet, sour, or salty taste. These foods, as well as foods that are cold or oily, are Kapha-increasing; they have a tendency to both increase mucus production and constrict the sinus passages. With a buildup of mucus and a blockage of the sinuses, the chances for infection are greatly increased.

To prevent colds and sinus problems and to treat them effectively if they arise, you need to eat a balanced diet and cut down on congestion-producing foods. How much of each taste you require in your personal diet will depend on your body type.

If you are a Vata type, you can get away with a substantial amount of sweet, sour, and salty food without any ill effects. These three tastes are actually balancing and good for you. However, even for you, too much is too much—if you tend to get colds, take a look at your diet first, and if you're eating too many Kapha-increasing foods, cut back.

Pittas can handle a low to moderate amount of sour and salty, and quite a bit of sweet. If you are a Kapha body type, however, you will have to limit your intake of these three tastes.

THE HOT WATER CURE

One valuable, extremely simple, and absolutely free technique to ward off colds is to drink a few sips of hot water frequently throughout the day. Do this if you feel a cold coming on and you will be very pleased by the effect.

If you are prone to colds or sinus problems, I suggest that you make a habit of sipping an ounce or two—or more if you like—of hot water every half hour or so. (You can carry a thermos with you to work.) This is a safe and simple way to reduce Kapha and ama (impurity) in the body.

If you do come down with a cold or your sinuses become congested, immediately cut down on sweets, particularly foods containing refined sugar, and reduce consumption of salty foods such as chips, which also have the Kapha-increasing quality of being oily. Favor foods that tend to reduce congestion, such as soups and other warm or hot liquids, steamed or lightly sauteed vegetables, whole grains, and drier (less oily) foods, which are usually in the bitter, pungent, and astringent taste categories.

When you have a cold, or if you tend to get colds often, take suggestions from the Kapha-pacifying diet in Chapter 3. Even if you don't have a Kapha body type, if you tend toward colds you may be eating too many Kapha-increasing foods, such as red meat, foods rich in wheat or dairy (especially cheese, milk, and yogurt), fried or oily foods, and too much candy, pastry, or other sweets. These will tend to build up excess Kapha if you don't eat them in moderation. This was a main part of Jennifer's problem, and cutting down on these foods was extremely helpful to her.

If you have a Kapha constitution and tend to have a lot of colds, you need to follow the Kapha diet guidelines more conscientiously.

Eating a very light diet, mostly made up of thin (noncreamy) soups, will help reduce the production of mucus. If you feel a cold coming on, eat lightly like this for a few days. It's also important not to eat if you don't feel hungry. Eating three meals a day out of habit, even when your body doesn't send you the signal to eat, will increase your chances of developing colds or sinus problems.

Additional Strategies for Preventing Colds

Although a light, Kapha-pacifying diet may cure your cold, some other techniques and strategies are often helpful. These reduce the cold-producing risk factors such as irritation and dryness and strengthen digestive power.

Reduce Dryness to Protect Your Sinuses

John, 66, had lived most of his life in the Midwest. As he got older, he found that his Vata constitution made him feel increasingly uncomfortable in the cold winters. When he and his wife retired, they made a move to Arizona, to escape the winter temperatures.

John liked the warmth of Arizona, but the dryness disagreed with him. He found that his sinuses were almost always blocked, and he developed several sinus infections as a result. The nasal sprays his doctor prescribed helped for a while, but they stopped working after a week or so. The allergy pills he took were making him drowsy. After getting an Ayurvedic consultation, he was advised to do a few simple things to reduce dryness, and lo and behold, his sinuses got better. Here are the suggestions:

- Dip your little finger in some sesame oil and insert the tip of the finger inside each nostril. Sniff, then gently massage the mucous membrane with your finger. Repeat this procedure two or three times during the day. This will keep the sinuses and nasal passages from drying up and will also serve as a barrier against infections. (If the prospect of using your finger to do this procedure is disturbing, use a nose dropper. Squeeze in two or three drops, then sniff.)
- Put five drops of Vata aroma oil* into an electric crock pot filled three-fourths full with water and turn on the pot. Keep the door closed to keep the moist air from escaping. The Vata-balancing herbs combined with the moisture will reduce the tendency toward dryness. Even without the oil, prudent use of a vaporizer or humidifier will help.

Following these suggestions should also reduce your susceptibility to allergies.

Keep Your Digestion Strong

Improper eating habits that weaken the body's digestive ability are one of the most common causes of colds and sinus congestion. As mentioned earlier, overeating, and eating too fast, both tend to produce ama. This partially digested food eventually becomes toxic and leads to disease. So slow down, chew your food thoroughly, and try not to overeat. This will permit complete digestion and prevent the buildup of congestion.

---

*Available in some natural food stores or from MAPI products; see Appendix C.

Another key to preventing colds is to keep the body's digestive fire or *agni* lively. In Chapter 10 I will explain several ways for you to keep the fires burning brightly so that your digestive furnace can make maximum use of your food. Among these are adequate exercise, good eating habits, eating your main meal at midday, and eating food that stimulates the digestive system, such as pungent or spicy food, in appropriate amounts for your constitution.

One simple way to keep your digestion efficient is to start meals with a pinch or two of ginger pickle:

GINGER PICKLE

Grate a small amount of fresh ginger root. Add to that a little fresh lemon juice and a pinch of salt. A few minutes before you start eating, eat a pinch or two of this rather hot concoction to get your digestive juices flowing.

It is not an exaggeration to say that every item of food, and how we eat it, has an effect on our health. Since we have complete control over these factors, preventing and treating colds (and many other health problems, too) is largely within our grasp.

Be Sure to Get Your Immunity Boosters

Strengthening digestion in itself helps to strengthen immunity, as does regular exercise. In addition, there are a variety of natural substances that for centuries have been known to improve immune functioning, which in turn should help to prevent colds.

In Ayurveda these herbal and fruit mixtures are called *rasayanas,* formulas that promote health in all the body's organs and tissues, thereby strengthening our overall resistance to disease. These immunity boosters are said to enhance not only physical but also psychological immunity. Recent research has shown the validity of these ancient formulas.*

These immunity boosters can be found in most natural food stores:

---

*For example, see the work of Hari Sharma, M.D., of Ohio State University.

- *Triphala:* A combination of three potent Ayurvedic herbs
- *Maharishi Amrit Kalash:* An ancient herbal formula found by recent research to strengthen immunity. (Using both the "Ambrosia" tablets and "Nectar" jam creates a complete rasayana.)
- *Chyavanprash:* A traditional Ayurvedic formula based on the *amalak* fruit, which is extremely high in vitamin C.
- *Ginger:* Use in cooking, or see recipe for ginger tea in next section.

Taking any of these herbal preparations daily should help prevent colds. Take the products as directed on labels.

Head Off Colds by Living in Tune with Mother Nature

Another important factor in whether or not we come down with colds is how we interact with the natural environment. Ayurveda traditionally teaches that the weather, for example, can strongly influence our health.

Watch the Weather

The windy and cold weather characteristic of fall and winter can debilitate our immune system and create problems in the nose and sinus cavities if we don't respond intelligently to those conditions. So that advice our mothers gave us—"Don't forget to wear your hat"—may turn out to be right after all. Swimming in cold water, drinking ice-cold drinks, not covering our face and ears in windy weather all make us prone to catching a cold.

The weather in the late fall, winter, and early spring increases Vata and Kapha, the two main culprits in developing a cold. The mostly windy, wet, and cold character of these seasons tends to

- slow down digestion, resulting in increased mucus accumulation;
- constrict the sinus passages, increasing the chance of blockage by the accumulated mucus—perfect conditions for bacteria and virus growth;
- irritate the mucous membranes, resulting in a breakdown of the body's natural barrier against infections.

You need to protect yourself from the influence of these environmental conditions in order to prevent a cold from developing. Wear a hat, scarf, gloves, and a warm coat in cold weather. This is especially important for Vata and Kapha constitutions. Pittas may generate enough internal heat to need less wrapping-up. (That's why some people can get away with wearing only a jacket when others are shivering under their heavy coats.)

Staying warm and protected will definitely help to prevent the onset of a cold. Again, drinking hot water at intervals during the day keeps the body warm internally, opens the sinus passages, and serves as a good prevention technique.

Eating foods that reduce Vata in the fall, and Kapha in the winter and spring is also helpful. (Please refer to the food charts in Chapter 3.) Warm, well-cooked foods that are on the spicy side are more beneficial during these "cold-prone" seasons.

Get enough rest

As was the case with Jennifer, whose story opened this chapter, tiredness due to insufficient sleep at night weakens the immune system. A strong immune system is our primary line of defense against colds (see Chapter 5). So getting to bed in time to get a good night's rest is a very important choice we can make to help us avoid getting sick.

Warm up colds with exercise

Keeping the internal heat of the body higher through regular, appropriate exercise is another important way to increase immunity and decrease the tendency toward congestion in colder weather. The word "appropriate" is important here. Both overexercise and underexercise can give rise to colds.

Overexercising is tiring to the body, and fatigue tends to reduce immunity. On the other hand, underexercising lets digestion get sluggish, which disallows effective cleansing of mucus and other impurities from the digestive system. So it's important to find the happy medium, the type and amount of exercise that is right for you. As you learned in Chapter 7, this varies for each body type.

GINGER TEA: AN EFFECTIVE COLD REMEDY

Ginger tea is warming and drying and helps to immediately reduce the symptoms of a cold.

You can easily make your own ginger tea. Pick up some ginger root in your natural food store or the produce department of your local supermarket. (Don't let the price-per-pound scare you; you need only a few ounces.) Take a small piece (weighing about an ounce), peel, and slice thinly. Place in a quart of water, cover, and boil until the water is about half gone. (This will make a pretty snappy-tasting tea.) When the tea is still warm but has cooled down enough to drink, add 1/2 to 1 full teaspoon of honey to your cup. Be sure not to heat the honey too much; it becomes less digestible when heated. And don't feel guilty for using a sweetener. Honey is the only sweetener that has a drying effect and is excellent for reducing Kapha.

You can drink several cups of ginger tea each day for as long as your cold lasts. It is also useful for reducing Kapha when taken on a regular basis.

Herbal Cold Remedies

Herbs can be effective both in preventing and treating colds. Here are a few that may be helpful:

Ginger
Ginger contains all six tastes and therefore is very nourishing to the whole system. As mentioned earlier, it is one of the category of herbs known in Ayurveda as rasayanas, or revitalizers.

In addition to its immune-enhancing property, ginger is also spicy and tends to reduce mucus and congestion in the upper respiratory system. (All spicy-type foods and herbs are Kapha reducing.) To prevent or treat a cold, ginger can be taken as a tea or as tablets, both readily available in natural food stores.

Turmeric
Available in natural food stores and in almost all groceries in the spice section,* turmeric is famous in Ayurveda for its Kapha-

---

*Try to buy turmeric in bulk in a natural food store. It is liable to be fresher and much less expensive than in the small bottles or tins in grocery stores.

IF YOU HAVE A REALLY BAD COLD . . .

Ayurvedic approaches to preventing and treating colds are effective and often work without the need for any Western medicines. The Ayurvedic approach is especially helpful in the prevention and early treatment of a developing cold.

However, there are occasions when a secondary bacterial infection may set in, especially when preventive or early treatment measures weren't taken. If fever develops, or yellow or green mucus appears, see a medical doctor. (It's ideal if your Western-trained doctor is also versed in Ayurveda, but this isn't always possible.) If the doctor prescribes an antibiotic, or any other medications, you may continue with the Ayurvedic recommendations at the same time. This should speed up the recovery as well as prevent relapses.

reducing properties. This is because it is strongly astringent in taste and tends to dry up the mucous membranes. Using turmeric with your food (it's the yellow color in curry) and also taking 1/4 to 1/2 teaspoon with about a teaspoon of honey 2–3 times a day can be helpful in reducing congestion.

Black pepper
Adding some extra black pepper to your food will also help to reduce congestion.

In general, all the pungent herbs, which reduce Kapha, are helpful in preventing and treating colds. These include black pepper, celery seed, cloves, cumin, mustard seed, chili peppers, cayenne, and ginger.

When a cold strikes, Western medicine has powerful medicines that can provide dramatic symptom relief. But if you really want to have a life free of runny noses, coughing, cold sores, sinus headaches, and the whole constellation of cold symptoms, the best thing to do is structure a way of life that will build your immunity and keep your body in balance. Ayurveda, the ancient health science rooted in nature, provides ready, time-tested guidelines.

CHAPTER 10

TUNE UP YOUR DIGESTION

From ancient times until today, Ayurvedic physicians have emphasized the importance of digestion in maintaining good health, a clear mind, and balanced emotions. In fact, Ayurveda teaches that how well you digest is even more important than what you actually eat.

Even the best of foods, if inadequately digested, won't get properly absorbed into the body. When digestion is incomplete, the partially digested food is not only relatively useless for nourishment, but can also accumulate in the intestines and become the cause of illness. That's why, in addition to specific recommendations about what to eat, Ayurveda has many suggestions about how to prepare your food and how to eat it, in order to keep digestion working at maximum efficiency.

We will explore these important suggestions in this chapter.

Light Up Your Digestive Fire

The key to complete, healthy digestion is called *agni,* or the "digestive fire." Of course, agni is not conceived as a literal fire; it is the overall name for the enzymes, acids, and biochemistry of the stomach and intestines that break down the food and prepare it for assimilation. When the digestive fire is strong, digestion is efficient and complete. Foods are fully broken down and metabolized, bringing nourishment to all the body's cells and tissues.

Ayurveda distinguishes four states of agni:

Balanced

Due to a balance of the three doshas (Vata, Pitta, and Kapha), it results in healthy digestion and assimilation and is characterized by comfortable digestion, regular bowel movements, energy, mental clarity, and an overall sense of cheerfulness and interest in life and work.

Diminished

In general, Kapha digestion tends to be slow. Diminished digestive fire is generally due to a Kapha imbalance (excess Kapha in the system) and results in heaviness, sluggishness, and a tendency toward overweight.

Excess

The digestion of people with Pitta body types tends to be intense and strong. Too much Pitta in the system results in a voracious appetite and eating large amounts of food, but paradoxically there may be weakness or emaciation caused by the body's "burning up" the food before it can be absorbed.

Irregular

This is usually due to too much Vata in the system, resulting in fluctuations in appetite, inconsistent ability to digest food, and typical Vata digestive disorders such as gas, constipation, or diarrhea. Vata body types have rather delicate digestive systems that are more easily thrown off and upset than the other two types.

When digestion is incomplete or ineffective due to an imbalance in one of the doshas, health can be seriously weakened. Here is a description of what happens when food remains only partially digested, as explained by one of the world's leading Ayurvedic physicians, Dr. Vasant Lad:

> Food components remain undigested and unabsorbed. They accumulate in the large intestine turning into a heterogeneous, foul-smelling, sticky substance. This material, which is called *ama,* clogs the intestines and other channels, such as capillaries and blood vessels. It eventually undergoes many chemical changes which create toxins.

These toxins are absorbed into the blood and enter the general circulation. They eventually accumulate in the weaker parts of the body, where they create contraction, clogging, stagnation and weakness of the organs and reduce the immune mechanism of the respective tissues. Finally, a disease condition manifests in the affected organs.

Though Western medicine does not have an exact parallel to ama, many diseases are known to result from the accumulation of metabolic wastes resulting from poor digestion. Several examples, from among many pointed out by the authors of *A Woman's Best Medicine: Health, Happiness and Long Life Through Maharishi Ayur-Veda*, include the following:

- "Bad" LDL cholesterol is a sticky substance that accumulates in the arteries and may lead to stroke and heart attack.
- Undigested fats can produce blockages resulting in eye disease and cirrhosis of the liver.
- Underdigested carbohydrates can cause diabetes.

The key to healthy digestion thus is to maintain the agni, or digestive fire, at a high level of efficiency.

WATCH OUT FOR AMA

The product of partially or inadequately digested food is called ama. This is a sticky, foul-smelling substance that clogs up the body's inner channels and leads to disease. Some of the signs that there is ama in the body include:

- dull eyes or skin
- coated tongue in the morning; unpleasant taste in the mouth
- bad breath
- cloudy or discolored urine
- weak digestion
- chronic diarrhea or constipation
- loss of appetite

Six Factors for Getting the Most Nourishment from Your Food

The following suggestions aim at keeping your digestive fires burning brightly so that you can gain maximum benefits from the food you eat. Except where otherwise stated, these recommendations are for all constitutional types.

What Foods Should You Eat?

In addition to eating foods that are proper for your body type and appropriate for the season, keep the following tips in mind concerning what you eat:

- Food should be fresh and natural, as free from artificial chemicals such as pesticides and fertilizers as possible. Avoid leftovers and all foods that are old, spoiled, burnt, stale, overcooked, etc.
- Use the best quality food you can afford. After all, "you are what you eat." You are a quality person, and you deserve quality food.
- Favor cooked food over raw. Cooked food (and Ayurveda suggests that food be cooked quite thoroughly) is easier to digest. Fruit is an exception and should form a significant part of your diet. Salads of raw vegetables do not play a large role in traditional Ayurvedic cuisine, but are acceptable, especially for Pittas whose strong digestive fire can handle the challenge. The roughage does serve as an aid to digestion when you eat a salad as a supplement to the main course. If you are a Vata type, be sure to include an oily dressing with your salad.
- Don't heat honey very much; never bake with it. According to Ayurveda, honey becomes hard to digest when heated more than enough to make it flow.
- Milk should be taken separately from a major meal, but combines well with grains, including cereals. Milk is best consumed heated. To improve digestibility, add a pinch of turmeric, ginger powder, or cardamom. A little honey (added after the milk is cool enough to drink) or raw sugar can be added.

- For all constitutions except Pitta, it is helpful to start each meal—particularly your heaviest meal of the day—with a ginger pickle (see recipe on p. 142) or chew a small amount of fresh ginger. This stimulates the digestive juices. (Pittas may find the ginger too heating.)
- In the evening, avoid heavy and Kapha-producing foods such as cheese, yogurt, buttermilk, and ice cream, which are difficult to digest and tend to produce ama.
- Avoid ice-cold food and drink. These impede and impair digestion. In Ayurvedic terms, their coldness tends to put out the digestive fire.
- Fried food is hard for your digestive enzymes to break down. It should be eaten only occasionally and by those whose digestive fire is strong.
- In general, lean toward a vegetarian diet. Meats are heavy and hard to digest, and they putrefy quickly in the digestive tract, producing ama.

In the food charts in Chapter 3, acceptable meats for each body type are listed. You may eat them in small quantities, if you wish. But if you eat all six tastes there should be no need for meat in order to fulfill your protein requirement.

Modern medical research now has significant evidence that a balanced vegetarian diet may be the most healthful. According to the American Dietetic Association, the main professional organization of registered dieticians:

> A considerable body of scientific data suggests positive relationships between vegetarian lifestyles and risk reduction for several chronic degenerative diseases and conditions, such as obesity, coronary artery disease, hypertension, diabetes mellitus, colon cancer, and others. . . . Vegetarians also have lower rates of osteoporosis, lung cancer, breast cancer, kidney stones, gallstones, and diverticular disease.

Need I say more in support of reducing your meat intake?

When reducing meat in the diet (or making any other major dietary changes), it is usually best to do so *gradually,* to allow the system to adjust comfortably, rather than by going "cold turkey," which can be too much of a strain.

There's a bonus for following these Ayurvedic guidelines for healthy digestion. By eating less fried food and less or no fatty meat, cutting down on heavy foods at night, and so on, and by keeping your digestive fires strong instead of sluggish, you will almost automatically avoid being overweight. And as you know, being overweight is itself a major risk factor in many serious diseases including hypertension, heart disease, gall bladder disease, and adult onset diabetes.

How Should the Food Be Prepared?

Ayurveda places great emphasis on the quality of the person who prepares and cooks the food. The thoughts and feelings of the cook affect the food and later affect the eater of the food. If a person cooks while feeling anger, fear, resentment, sadness, those qualities get transmitted and are absorbed by the eater. As Ayurvedic physician Robert Svoboda writes,

> Ideally, your food should be grown in your own field or garden so that you have full control over what physical and mental inputs it imbibes. . . . Every thought thought by the cook affects the food and, after ingestion, the eater. Only one who loves you and is ready to devote the effort needed to transmit that love into the food should cook for you.

Obviously, this principle also applies to you when you cook for others. Choosing fine-quality foods and preparing them with love is nourishing on every level. Perhaps that is why, when young students used to question a famous Indian teacher about what they should eat, his first reply would be, "Eat whatever Mother puts on the table."

When to Eat

As mentioned in the chapter on the ideal daily routine, it is best to eat the heaviest meal of the day at noon, when the agni, or digestive fire, is strongest. Supper should be light and eaten at least two hours before going to bed. Breakfast is optional, depending on your hunger level and body type, as the following points will indicate:

- **Pittas** generally require three meals a day and sometimes need snacks in between, but they should leave a gap of at least three or four hours in between. A good snack for Pittas is sweet fruit, such as grapes, peaches, or mangoes. Also, dried fruits such as dates and raisins are good. A common cause of irritability for people with a Pitta constitution is missing a meal, especially lunch. Pitta people are often very ambitious and thus have important and high-pressure jobs; they may easily find themselves in a situation where it's difficult to eat lunch or to take enough time to eat it properly. They need to guard against this. It can result not only in irritability, but in hyper-acidity, skin rashes, ulcers, and other Pitta disorders.

- **Kapha** types often prefer to skip breakfast, and that is right and good for them. They shouldn't feel they have to eat three meals a day as we in the West have been cultured to believe. Kaphas tend not to feel hungry. If they go ahead and eat anyway, ignoring this natural inclination, they'll easily become overweight and will probably feel sluggish and depressed. Kaphas should leave at least six hours between meals and are better off if they don't snack in between, so that digestion can be completed.

- **Vatas** have a tendency to eat irregularly, but it is very balancing for them to eat at regular times during the day. Most authorities suggest that Vatas eat at least three or even four light (i.e., small) meals a day, with snacks in between as desired. A gap of at least two hours between meals and/or snacks is a minimum. Vatas should respect the variability of their appetite, which is normal for their constitution, but should make an effort to eat on schedule. This will help dispel nervousness, restlessness, anxiety, insomnia, spaciness, nervous depression, and other Vata problems.

- After eating, all body types should wait at least an hour before beginning any strenuous exercise, though a short walk after meals can help digestion. The traditional Ayurvedic literature suggests a "stroll of 100 steps."

- Though it is good to follow a regular schedule for meals, the key principles to follow about timing are these: The right time to eat is when you're hungry; the wrong time is when you're not. The right time to eat is when you can be relaxed and settled. The wrong time to eat is when you're rushed.

How Much Should You Eat?

The stomach has difficulty digesting if it is too full. Follow these guidelines to gauge how much is enough, and try not to overeat.

- Eat only to about 2/3 or 3/4 of your capacity, so that you feel satisfied but not stuffed.
- A traditional Ayurvedic formula is to fill your stomach 1/3 with food and 1/3 with liquid, leaving 1/3 empty for ease of digestion.
- A good rule of thumb is to eat approximately the quantity of food that you could hold by cupping your two hands together.
- One helpful way to tell if you are full or not is to put a hand over the stomach area in order to better focus your attention on the digestive process.

Improving Your Eating Environment

True to Ayurveda's holistic perspective on life, this ancient science teaches that the nature of your surroundings during meals influences the effects of the food on your digestion and absorption.

Just think about it for a minute: Where do you think you would feel more comfortable eating, in a hot, noisy, crowded cafeteria with bare tables and busboys rolling carts full of clattering dishes and silverware—or in a quiet, settled restaurant with tablecloths, flowers on the table, soft music playing . . . ?

It's obvious, yet most of us rarely take the time to set up a congenial environment for our meals. Try it; your digestive system will be as glad as you are.

Enjoy the Process

In addition to creating a comfortable, peaceful environment for your meals, there are many other ways to enhance the enjoyment of eating and increase the efficiency of digestion.

- Eat sitting down, in a nonhurried fashion.
- Before you eat, have a moment of silence or say a brief prayer of thanks for the food. This helps you relax and sets the stage for better digestion.

- Pay attention to what you're doing, which is a rather sacred task: converting elements of the environment into you, so that you can be creative and of service to others. Avoid distractions such as TV or reading. These tend to divert blood flow from the stomach, resulting in indigestion and inadequate assimilation.
- Chew your food well until it's soft. A trick to help you do this is to put your fork down between bites and lift it up only after each mouthful has been fully chewed and swallowed.
- Avoid stress or tension during a meal. Try not to talk about overdue bills, conflicts at work, or other emotional issues. Also, it's best not to eat at all if you are feeling angry, depressed, or otherwise emotionally overwhelmed. This is very important, because you absorb along with the food whatever feelings you are feeling while you eat.
- Sit at least five minutes after a meal before getting up.
- After eating, take a short walk as suggested above. Or lie down for a few minutes, preferably on your left side.

If you combine the suggestions in this chapter with the more comprehensive recommendations for *what* to eat and *when* to eat it, contained in Chapters 3 and 6, you will have a complete formula for lifelong healthful eating.

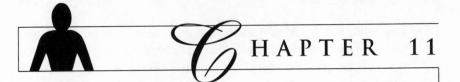

CHAPTER 11

How to Achieve Your Ideal Weight

Nearly every morning Marie looked at herself in the mirror and felt a sinking feeling in her stomach. Her fleshy arms, heavy breasts, and rounded belly just didn't look like the models in the magazines or the actresses on TV, those women with the long, thin limbs who had what Marie felt was an ideal body. She wanted to look like that too.

Of course, she had *never* looked anything like that. From the time she was a young child, she had always been one of the larger, heavier girls.

On the other hand, everyone told Marie that she was not fat. Her doctor repeatedly assured her that her weight was completely in the normal range. "You've simply got a larger frame," he said. Her friends told her she was a "beautiful, curvaceous woman," and men seemed to find her attractive. The only problem was her own attitude. She felt fat, and that feeling gnawed at her self-esteem.

Marie's dilemma may sound familiar to you. At any one time in America, approximately 50 million people are on a diet, and about 75 percent of American women—three out of every four—think they need to lose weight. But how many of them *really* need to?

Certainly there are people who are overweight and ought to take off some pounds for health reasons. But many of the others are just suffering from "image-itis"—they have an idealized image of beauty, based on what they see in the media, and they are suffering because they don't live up to that image.

156

Ayurveda has a simple and clear response to this dilemma, an explanation and a solution based on the fundamental principle of different body types. The explanation is that—in case you haven't noticed—people naturally come in all shapes and sizes. We are all different, and that difference is due to our constitutional type. Some people will naturally be thin. That is their body type, by birth. Such people can eat and eat, and chances are they won't gain any weight at all.

Marie envied her friend Janet, the possessor of one of those thin, petite bodies. But one day Janet told her, "I'm so flat-chested and bony; I'm sick of looking at my ribs and my hip bones. I'd give *anything* to be built more like you, but I just can't seem to put on any weight."

Other people, like Marie, will naturally be heavier. This is *their* body type. These people feel that they gain weight if they just *think* about eating, and indeed, they do have a tendency to put on the pounds if they don't keep themselves in balance. But no matter how hard they work at keeping slim, they will always have a larger frame and tend toward a stockier, fuller build than those who are constitutionally thin.

The solution is just as simple as the explanation: Each type is normal, healthy, and beautiful when mind and body are in balance. So whatever you are, whatever Mother Nature has designed for you, embrace it and enjoy it. Just as it's not any better to be a pine tree than an apple tree, it's not better, not healthier, not more beautiful to be born with a body that belongs to one type than another.

Thus the goal of this chapter is twofold. First, we are going to assess whether the weight you now are is actually—all idealized images aside—a normal, natural weight for you. If it is, I hope you will find enough support here to become comfortable with this weight and gain peace of mind about it for the rest of your life.

Second, if you discover that you *are* actually overweight—or underweight, for that matter—this chapter will give you many time-tested and effective suggestions for moving in the direction of the weight you want to be.

Overcoming Image-Itis

If you are an art lover, you know that artists in earlier times had images of ideal beauty quite different from today's ideal. The nineteenth-century painter Renoir comes to mind. His canvases depict lovely women, often painted nude, whose pink bodies would, by today's standards, be considered more than a little plump. But by the cultural standards of his time—less than 100 years ago in Europe—these women were ideal beauties.

As far as *you* are concerned, all these standards are irrelevant, whether they're the standards of Renoir's time, of *Playboy* or *Glamour* magazine, or any other external measure. And before we go any further, let's get clear that although the concern about body image or being overweight seems to be more prevalent among women, these statements are, of course, equally true for men. The muscular hunks who inhabit body-building magazines and ads for exercise equipment do not constitute an ideal model of manhood—unless you think they do.

If you are a Vata type, your chances of looking like a Renoir model or a *Playboy* centerfold are pretty thin—because *you* will be pretty thin. It is characteristic of Vatas to have smaller bones and lean bodies. A powerful, muscular male physique or a busty, curvaceous female form is something a Vata cannot realistically expect to see looking back from the mirror.

Vatas not only have no trouble losing weight, it is often a struggle for them to keep their weight up at a "normal" level. Vatas are thin as children and usually remain slender throughout their lives. They have small muscles and narrow chests, though Vata women sometimes have disproportionately large breasts on their slender frames.

These lean bodies may be the envy of people with the heavier, more solid frame typical of Kaphas. Kaphas are naturally bigger boned, with stronger, thicker muscles and broad shoulders and hips. Often plump as children, Kaphas put on weight easily all their lives and take it off only with effort. They are strong, well-proportioned, and move with grace.

In between the lean Vata and sturdy Kapha is the Pitta, whose body type is often described as "medium." The term is appropriate. Fiery, ambitious, intelligent Pittas tend to be of medium build (neither thin nor stocky), of medium height, and with medium-sized shoulders and hips. But they also tend to be quite muscular and strong. Pittas gain weight fairly easily—they have excellent appetites and like to eat—but they generally have strong will power and can shed the pounds quickly if they decide to.

Each of these body types is natural; none is better or worse than any other. And realistically speaking, what difference would it make? We don't flip through a body-type catalog before birth and order the kind we prefer, nor can we make exchanges now; we're simply born into one, and it's our challenge to bring out the potential for health and beauty in the body we inhabit.

Whatever your body type, the specific guidelines in this book can help you maintain balance, vitality, and joy of living.

Maybe You're Already at Your Ideal Weight

Now is the time for you to have a moment of truth with yourself. You have taken the body type questionnaire early in the book, and you've now read about a dozen chapters that have given you a pretty solid understanding of the different Ayurvedic body types. You're fairly certain what type you are. So what follows is the bottom line.

If you are predominantly a Vata, chances are that you will be relatively thin most of your life. It is possible for Vatas to become overweight from what we might call nervous eating—excessive eating from being very high-strung and anxious—and this happens sometimes. But it is the exception, and when such an overweight Vata gets back in balance, the weight drops off quite naturally with little effort as the body returns to its naturally leaner shape.

So if you are a Vata and are currently overweight, don't worry about losing weight. If you are very thin—a more likely situation for a Vata—the same advice applies. In both cases, just put your attention on balancing the Vata, which you can do by having a more regular schedule, eating the Vata-balancing diet (warm and heavier foods, emphasizing the sweet, sour, and salty tastes, etc.), doing a daily sesame oil massage, and engaging in regular mild exercise. Please review the chapters on diet, exercise, and daily routine for tips on balancing Vata, as well as Pitta and Kapha.

If you are predominantly Pitta, you will have a medium build most of your life. You will probably never become very thin, nor are you likely to become obese, though compulsive eating may drive your weight up. Pittas often do have very intense energy, which can lead to compulsive behavior of various kinds, such as being a workaholic, being unreasonably competitive or perfectionistic, and so forth. This may carry over into the sphere of eating.

The remedy, as with Vatas, is generally not to focus on weight loss, but simply on getting back into balance. For this, follow the guidelines for a Pitta-balancing lifestyle. Don't get overheated or eat much spicy or salty food. Stay away from alcoholic drinks. Avoid highly competitive sports. Enjoy activities such as swimming, skiing, noncompetitive golf, and bicycle touring.

Now, if you are a Kapha, the chances are that you will have a large build and will already have been struggling with your weight most of your life. The crucial issue for you is to understand that you will *always* have a larger build. That wispy ballerina's body is something you just won't have. (On the other hand, the Ayurvedic literature is full of references to the beauty and grace Kaphas *do* naturally tend to have.)

But having a larger build doesn't mean you need to be "fat," nor that you *are* fat. Nor does it give you an excuse for self-indulgent eating and piling on excess pounds. If you follow a healthful routine for your body type—the Kapha-balancing diet, more vigorous exercise than for the other two types, foods that are lighter and spicier, and so on—there is no need for you ever to become overweight.

So take a minute now and think about it. Are you at a healthful weight for your body type? Have your worries about being too fat been based more on an idealized image, rather than on health considerations? If so, this is a good time to let yourself off the hook—permanently.

However . . .

If You Are Overweight . . .

All this is not to say that actually being overweight is okay. Modern medicine has found it to be a serious health concern, and Ayurveda has described it and treated it as a health problem for thousands of years. Charaka, one of the great ancient Ayurvedic physicians, pointed out quite clearly more than 3,000 years ago that obesity results in premature aging, a shorter life, reduced sexual drive and performance, difficulty in breathing and shortness of breath, excessive sweating, unpleasant body odor, tiredness, weakness, loss of vitality, and mental dullness and confusion.

Being overweight also leads to a number of serious diseases. Modern medicine has discovered this connection to other illnesses, but thousands of years ago Ayurvedic physicians noted many, including diabetes, arthritis, heart disease, high blood pressure (hypertension), menstrual disorders, kidney infections, and numerous others.

Dr. Subash Renade, an internationally known authority on Ayurveda, says that the main causes of obesity, not surprisingly, have to do with faulty diet and digestion. Particularly, they are a weakening of the digestive fire, production of ama or impurities due to improperly digested food, and a diet incompatible with one's body type. Other possible causal factors include inadequate exercise, sleeping during the day, and hereditary factors.

Seven Secrets to Losing Weight

The way to shed excess weight is based on counterbalancing these causal factors. Here's how to do it.

Stimulate your digestion

Chapter 10 provides dozens of suggestions for improving digestion. Several that are particularly helpful for encouraging weight loss:

- Sip hot water throughout the day.
- Fast one day a week on liquids. You may have fruit or vegetable juices, warm skim milk, light soups, teas, etc.
- Drink ginger tea 2–3 times per day.
- Use herbs and spices that are primarily pungent (spicy), bitter, or astringent. Common spices such as cumin, ginger, mustard seed, cayenne, and black pepper are helpful when used in cooking, or you can use Ayurvedic herbs such as *gotu kola, amalaki,* and *shilajit* in powder or capsule form. These herbs are available at many natural food stores or from the sources listed in Appendix C.
- Chew a thin slice of fresh ginger root a few minutes before meals to get the digestive juices flowing. Or grate a little ginger, mix with some lemon juice and salt, and eat a pinch or two.
- Exercise regularly according to your body type.

Eliminate ama

All the above measures for stimulating the digestive process are also effective for reducing ama, which by definition is a by-product of inefficient or incomplete digestion. Ama, as we saw in Chapter 5, is a sticky substance that is considered in Ayurveda to be a major causative factor in many, if not most, diseases. Much like cholesterol—which may someday be identified as a form of ama—it tends to clog up the circulatory, lymph, and other channels of the body. People who are overweight almost always have an excess of ama in their bodies.

According to Deepak Chopra, M.D.:

> It is highly impractical to treat any imbalance of the physiology when ama is present—and it is extremely difficult, perhaps impossible, to lose weight. This is why so many people who have limited their diets to the point of virtual starvation still have failed to accomplish their goals. Therefore it's essential to take practical steps to eliminate ama in order to lose weight and keep it off permanently. Ama is, quite simply, a key in the pathogenesis of obesity. After all, one of the principal qualities of ama is *heaviness*.

Here are a few more herbs and compounds that are effective in reducing ama: the common herbs turmeric and barberry, and the Ayurvedic herbal compounds *trikatu* (a combination of equal parts of black pepper, ginger, and *pippali* or Indian long pepper, which can be taken in capsule form to strengthen digestion and burn away ama); and *triphala* (a combination of *amalaki*, *bibhitaki*, and *haritaki*), which is said to scrape ama from the digestive tract and facilitate elimination. Both of these herbal compounds can be obtained very inexpensively (see Appendix C).

The Ayurvedic herb *guggulu* may also be helpful in facilitating fat metabolism and can be taken in combination with triphala.

What to eat

In most cases your weight problem will be connected to excess Kapha, and you will need to follow a Kapha-reducing diet. (It is possible, however, that your excess weight is due to an imbalance in either Vata or Pitta, or that an imbalance in one of these is "leading" the system to produce a Kapha imbalance. That is why it is always wise to consult an Ayurvedic practitioner for a diagnosis and advice whenever possible before beginning your self-healing program.)

In most cases it will be safe and helpful to follow a Kapha-reducing regimen. Detailed guidelines for the Kapha-balancing diet appear in Chapter 3 and center around lightening up your diet. This does not necessarily mean eating less (although that may be important for you) but rather, eating foods that are light rather than heavy, dry rather than moist, and that emphasize the pungent, astringent, and bitter tastes. Here are some good foods for Kapha reduction and weight loss:

Fruit Apples, pears, pomegranates, cranberries, cherries, most berries.

Vegetables Leafy green vegetables are good, such as spinach, beet greens, mustard greens, etc.

Dairy Avoid all dairy products as far as possible, except for occasional use of ghee. Use skim or low-fat milk.

Grains Basmati rice, barley, corn, millet, rye, and buckwheat are all acceptable.

Sweeteners Use only honey. Stay completely away from white sugar and all products containing white sugar.

Beverages As much as possible, restrict your drinking to warm or hot water. You can make a wide variety of herb teas with the warm water, or put half to one teaspoon of honey in the water once or twice a day (when the water is at a drinkable temperature).

Beans All beans are okay; red lentils and mung beans are excellent. Tofu is an excellent source of protein.

Spices All spices are okay, but especially pungent ones such as cayenne, black pepper, ginger, are recommended. Turmeric is also good. Salt is generally not recommended, but if you can get rock salt, that is okay.

What not to eat

It is equally important to avoid certain foods. In general, stay away from oily or greasy food, cold or iced food and drink, and minimize foods with sweet, sour, and salty taste.

Dairy: Avoid most dairy foods, especially cream, butter, cheese, and yogurt. Ice cream and other sweets made from both milk products and sugar are particularly off your list.

Grains: Avoid wheat products, including breads, cakes, and cookies. Other grains to minimize are oats and large amounts of rice. The current fad for oatmeal is not for you.

Fruit: Minimize sweet fruits such as avocado, coconut, dates, figs, grapes, pineapple, melons.

Vegetables: You'll do better without juicy vegetables such as yellow or zucchini squash, tomato, cucumber, and sweet potatoes.

Sweeteners: Honey is the only acceptable sweetener for you.

Nuts: Avoid all nuts—they're too oily and are usually salted.

Meats: A vegetarian diet is highly recommended, but if you eat meat, stay away from beef, and pork. Some chicken and fish are acceptable.

Beverages: Avoid all alcoholic drinks, including beer and wine. Keep away from carbonated drinks and other sweetened beverages. In general, avoid all cold and iced drinks.

When to eat

Rule number one here is: Eat only when you are hungry. If you're not hungry, even if it's your usual mealtime, don't eat. Your body will let you know when it needs food.

We have previously discussed another helpful choice you can make to ensure the most efficient, strongest digestion: Eat your largest, heaviest meal of the day at noon. This is the time when the agni or digestive fire is strongest.

Supper should be a lighter meal and is best eaten at least a couple of hours before you go to bed. Breakfast is optional depending on your hunger level, but in general it is not recommended for Kaphas, as they really don't need it.

Before You Eat . . .

Sit comfortably and close your eyes. You may say a brief prayer or just have a moment of silence. You can use this moment to give thanks for the food, but it also serves a couple of other important purposes. First, it gets you more in touch with yourself, with your hunger level now, so you'll know how much to eat; by maintaining that awareness, you will have less tendency to overeat.

Second, being quiet, stepping out of the whirlwind for a few seconds, is relaxing; it settles you down so you won't eat too fast. It will also help you avoid nervous or compulsive eating. If you have a problem with these issues, try just sitting quietly for a moment. You might find yourself feeling, "I'm not really hungry right now. Maybe I'll wait for half an hour and see if I'm more hungry then. . . ."

How much to eat?

Although weight loss is certainly dependent on not overeating, you can eat a large quantity of the right foods (such as fresh vegetables and fruit, light grains) and not gain weight, or a small quantity of the wrong foods (beef, cream, rich desserts) and gain a lot. So quantity is not necessarily the issue.

On the other hand, digestion is far more efficient if you don't pack your stomach full to the top. Too full, it has trouble digesting and may create ama. Follow these guidelines to gauge how much is enough:

- Eat only until you feel about 2/3 to 3/4 full, to a point where you're satisfied; stop before you feel stuffed.
- Try this formula: Fill your stomach 1/3 with food, 1/3 with liquid, and leave 1/3 empty for ease of digestion.
- Eat approximately the amount of food that you could hold in your two cupped hands.
- Here's an easy way to help you gauge whether you're hungry or not before a meal and whether you are getting full and ought to quit during a meal. Place one hand lightly on your stomach, close your eyes for half a minute to a minute, and see how you feel. You'll be surprised at how this helps you put your attention on what's going on inside.

  This is so simple, but it is a powerful tool for weight management because it helps you be aware of your own hunger level. Look to yourself; listen to yourself. You'll learn better every day to gauge what is good for you.
- Here's an important point that comes from a Western perspective rather than from Ayurveda: In order to lose weight, you have to burn up more calories than you take in. In other

words, you need to consume fewer calories in the food you eat than you burn up in your daily activities.

It's like the principle of good budgeting, only in reverse: You need to spend more than you earn. The best way to do this is to limit your intake of high-calorie foods such as sweets; full-fat dairy products such as butter and cream; and meat, especially beef and pork. These foods are all taboo on the Kapha-balancing diet anyway.

Make Exercise Central to Your Weight-Loss Program

You need to accomplish this reverse economy not only by restricting your income (eating), but also by increasing your expenditures (rate of burning energy). If your metabolism is sluggish—a typical problem for Kaphas and for most people who are overweight—you need to perk it up.

A sedentary lifestyle leads almost inevitably to a slow metabolism and a buildup of fat. Exercise has the function not only of burning calories while you're exercising, but also of increasing your overall rate of metabolism so that even while you're doing quiet work your system will be more actively burning calories.

Here are three key principles about your exercise program:

1. *It should be regular.* That means at least three or four times a week. Every day is even better, so long as the exercise is not so strenuous that you need a day off to recover. That sort of exercise is not recommended anyhow, which leads to point number 2:

2. *It should be comfortable.* Exercise that causes you to strain is *not* recommended in Ayurveda. The goal is not to work yourself into exhaustion, but to tone the body, enliven the digestion, and facilitate the absorption of nutrients and elimination of toxins. Proper exercise should leave you with more energy and vitality, not more tired than when you started. But how do you know how much exercise is right for you?

3. *The type and amount of exercise should be suited to your body type.* Consult Chapter 7 for a complete understanding and to

select the appropriate level of exercise for you. For now, here are a few reminders:

Vatas need the least amount of exercise. Vata exercise should be of the mild variety, consisting of such things as walking or light hiking, swimming, yoga stretching, comfortable bicycling, and so on. Vatas tire easily and should not strain. Exhaustion throws Vata out of balance; unbalanced Vata increases anxiety, which can lead to nervous overeating. Too much exercise can also result in people with Vata body types becoming too thin. So curb your natural Vata enthusiasm and don't overdo it.

Kaphas need the most vigorous exercise. Their naturally slower metabolism and tendency to put on weight requires firing up the system to a higher level in order to keep it in balance. This is true for prevention and "routine maintenance" and it is also true when a problem of excess weight has developed. Kaphas can use a sustained period (20 to 30 minutes or more) of aerobic exercise pretty much every day.

But be careful if you haven't exercised in a long time, or if you are over 40. Before beginning any exercise program, it is prudent to consult a physician to determine your limits.

Healthy exercise and sports choices for Kaphas include aerobic dance, jogging, rope jumping, vigorous swimming or cycling, or any other activity that really gets the juices flowing.

Exercise for **Pittas** should be intermediate between the high level of exertion required by the Kapha physiology and the lower level recommended for Vatas. Pittas are naturally inclined toward exercise and in general are quite good at sports, so they have many choices. They need to look out for two problems, both of which can aggravate Pitta and lead to compulsive eating:

1. overheating due to too much exertion;
2. too much competitiveness. Pittas are prone to be very competitive; it will be healthier for them if they use exercise as a way of balancing, relaxing, and reducing stress.

Good exercises for Pitta include swimming, skiing, jogging, and mountain climbing.

Remember that two exercises recommended for all body types are walking and the Salutation to the Sun. (Sun Salutation instructions are on pages 99–101.)

What If You're Too Thin?

We've been focusing on problems of excess weight because it is an issue—whether real or imagined—for so many people. But what if you're too thin?

Jeff was always on the go. An independent computer consultant, he never seemed able to sit still. He was always jabbering on the phone, or racing to a client's company to work on their computer system. Up in the early morning hours, he would regularly run at least three or four miles before going to work. His daily schedule was very erratic, as he often worked late into the night trying to solve a client's problem.

Jeff ate a lot but never seemed to put on weight. As he moved into middle age and his friends steadily increased in girth, they said he was lucky to be so thin, but it made him insecure, especially when he compared himself to the popular images of macho men bulging with muscles.

It wasn't until he read a book on Ayurveda that he understood that he was a Vata, with a naturally lean body frame. But he also realized that some of the things he was doing aggravated the situation. For one thing, he saw that his long morning runs were probably too much exertion for him, and he gradually cut down. He also began turning down those all-night consulting jobs so he could get more regular sleep.

Jeff also realized that his attempt to follow the standard low-fat, low-cholesterol diet was probably ill advised for a Vata, and he replaced his usual spare, cold lunch at the salad bar with something warmer and more substantial, often at a favorite Italian restaurant. And he learned how to give himself an oil massage, which he did almost daily.

Within a year Jeff had gained nearly 15 pounds and although his thin frame would never look like Arnold Schwarzenegger's, he did begin to look more solid. He started to feel different, too, more genuinely energetic and at the same time more settled and focused, so he was able to accomplish a lot more.

If you feel you are underweight for your body type, the situation can generally be remedied by following a Vata-pacifying routine, as Jeff did. That would involve eating warm, heavier foods and leaning toward foods that are almost exactly opposite the recommendations in the Kapha-reducing, weight-loss diet. Remember: we're all different. Foods that are bad for some people may be exactly what you need.

Three Steps to Overcoming Food Cravings and Compulsive Eating

One frequent source of trouble for people who become overweight is compulsive eating based on food cravings. These cravings often arise because your body is not getting sufficient nutrition from the food you eat. The body feels that it is lacking something and sends the signal to eat more, even if you are already quite full.

Most of the time you can't tell what it is that's missing, so you may go for foods that are not especially good for you, including snack foods such as ice cream, potato chips, pastries, and so on. This creates more ama, which generates further imbalance. Here are three steps to help you eliminate food cravings.

Step 1
Eat foods of all six tastes at every meal.

According to Ayurveda, eating foods representing all six tastes (sweet, sour, salty, bitter, pungent, astringent) provides a complete complement of vitamins, minerals, proteins, carbohydrates, fats, and trace elements and also gives the body a feeling of satisfaction. Thus it is recommended that you include foods from all six tastes at every main meal. Here's a review of the six tastes to help you plan your meals:

> *Sweet:* all grains including rice, barley, wheat, and therefore bread, pasta; milk and most dairy products (some are sour); many fruits; all meats; sugar; honey
>
> *Sour:* citrus fruits, vinegar, cheese, yogurt, some fruits such as peaches, plums, and pineapples in their not-quite-ripe state; tomatoes
>
> *Salty:* all foods with salt

Bitter: green leafy vegetables such as spinach; bitter greens (romaine lettuce, endive); horseradish; turmeric

Pungent: spicy foods and seasonings of all types; onions, radishes, garlic, pepper, ginger, cumin, cayenne

Astringent: beans and lentils, pomegranates, cabbage, broccoli, foods that have a drying, lip-puckering effect

Step 2

Savor your food. Pay attention to the smells and tastes of the food, both before you eat and while eating. This will help to stimulate the digestive enzymes even before you swallow the food. Cravings often occur due to incomplete digestion, as the body is not assimilating the food properly and receiving all its nutrients.

Step 3

Carry healthful snacks with you to work or wherever you go. This way, if you get a craving to eat you can have something that is healthful and won't throw your system farther out of balance.

Take along some raisins, almonds, dried apricots, and the like. When you get hungry between meals, drink a cup of warm skim milk into which you can add a pinch of ginger or turmeric powder and half a teaspoon of honey. Or try a glass of warm water with a little lemon juice and honey. (Remember not to heat the honey beyond warm.) You can take these drinks with you in a thermos. Be prepared, so the vending machines don't get the better of you.

Additional tip: An inexpensive and easily available herb that can be helpful in healing cravings is *gotu kola*. In addition to its benefits for digestion, this herb is calming to the mind and nervous system and thus may be helpful in eliminating the emotional basis of some food cravings. You can use capsules or make a tea by mixing a small amount of gotu kola in warm water with a little honey a couple of times a day.

A Note About Dieting

You may have noticed that in this entire chapter on weight, we haven't mentioned dieting. That's because Ayurveda frowns on the process of going on a weight-loss diet. And wisely so: Statistics reveal that despite the billions of dollars Americans spend dieting, about 90 percent of people who diet return to their original weight or even higher. Worse, the process of depriving their bodies of nourishment often has negative effects on their overall health.

On the other hand, there is something you can do. Light fasting, consisting of skipping one or two evening meals per week or taking liquids only one day per week can be helpful in strengthening digestion, which should help reduce weight over time.

Ayurvedic authorities believe that the best way to lose weight, gain weight, or maintain a healthy weight is to keep your body in balance. That means to follow the lifestyle guidelines for your specific body type. When you eat the proper foods for you, meditate, exercise in an appropriate manner, and so forth, your body will naturally bring itself into balance without any need for drastic measures. And it will maintain that new, balanced, more healthy state over the long haul.

So let go of the idea of crash diets and quick weight loss; it's not good for you. Relax; rejoice in whatever body the good Lord gave you, and learn to treat it right, according to its nature. That's the royal road to perfect health and perfect weight.

Healthy Is Beautiful

Now, let's get philosophical for a moment and return to the issue that began this chapter: What is beautiful? Do we have to conform to a certain external standard? Or is beauty something else?

Could it be that our full, natural beauty is directly related to our state of mental and physical health? No matter how "pretty" someone's features may be, if that person is depressed, angry, bitter, then where is the beauty? On the other hand, someone without "perfect" features who exudes health, joy, and a kind of radiance from inside exhibits a great deal of beauty.

According to Ayurveda, that inner beauty associated with ideal health comes from ojas. We talked about ojas when we discussed immunity (in Chapter 5). It is a hormonelike substance produced by the body that nourishes and regulates the nervous system and all the other cells and tissues in the body as well. Ojas is like a superoil that supports the body to run at peak performance levels.

As ama is at the source of virtually all disease and creates weakness, dullness, fatigue, depression, and low immunity, ojas is at the source of health, vitality, happiness, brilliance of mind, and strength of body. A person with a high level of ojas is said to have a glowing, youthful, and beautiful appearance, reflecting an inner feeling of lightness, energy, and an overall feeling of well-being and joy.

As ama is the by-product of an imbalanced lifestyle including poor eating habits, lack of exercise, and so on, ojas is the result of living a healthy life. Lifestyle habits that increase ojas include appropriate exercise; eating a nutritious, tasty, well-balanced diet of fresh foods, preferably vegetarian; listening to beautiful music; regularly getting a good night's rest; enjoying one's work; daily oil massage; and being out as often as possible in beautiful places in nature, where we can be exposed to the sun, fresh air, trees, and bodies of water.

If we build our system of these elements and keep ourselves in balance, no matter what our body type may be, we will glow with health and beauty.

CHAPTER 12

OVERCOME INSOMNIA AND GET A GOOD NIGHT'S SLEEP

Rest is the basis of activity. You know this from your own experience. If you sleep well at night, you function well in the daytime. If you don't sleep well, you don't function up to par. Your reactions are slower, your mind feels heavy and dull, you tend to get upset more easily, you don't work as efficiently, and in general it's a lot harder to get through the day. The ancient Ayurvedic physician Charaka said,

> Happiness and misery, obesity and leanness, strength and weakness, sexual vigor and impotence, consciousness and loss of sensory acuity, even life and death, depend on the quality of sleep.

We all know we need to get a good night's sleep, yet today, as in all ages in the past, people sometimes have a hard time getting to sleep or staying asleep. We toss and turn, with all our responsibilities, worries, and decisions pressing on us; the more we toss and the later it gets, the more anxious we become about how we're going to get through the day.

Insomnia comes in three basic types: either we have trouble falling asleep, trouble staying asleep, with frequent awakenings

173

during the night, or we wake up early and just can't get back to sleep. All of these have the same fundamental effect: We fail to get the amount of sleep we need, so we're tired the next day.

Missing sleep is more than inconvenient. Recurrent insomnia can throw the whole system out of balance and can lead to chronic fatigue. Some researchers have made an association between insomnia and other diseases, such as depression and anxiety. So it's very important that we do whatever we need to do in order to sleep well.

Fortunately, this is an area in which Ayurvedic therapies can have outstanding results.

How Much Sleep Do You Really Need?

Before you decide that you have a problem with sleep, it might be valuable to consider how much sleep you really need. We've all heard the standard prescription—eight hours—but is that correct for everyone? Now that you've been studying Ayurveda, you're probably suspicious of a universal standard. What about the different body types? Don't people with different body types need different amounts of sleep?

The answer is yes, the requirements *are* different. The most sleep is needed by Kapha types, who generally require eight or nine hours in order to feel rested. Pittas are next, with a need of seven to eight hours. Vatas generally are content with six to seven hours.

But there's another consideration here, and that is, what stage of life are you in? Babies, as you know, can sleep as much as 15 or 16 hours out of every 24. Children frequently sleep 10 hours or more. At the other extreme, elderly people rarely enjoy a sound, unbroken sleep of more than four or five hours.

Interestingly, Ayurveda considers childhood to be the Kapha stage of life. Adulthood is Pitta time, and old age is the Vata stage of life. So the same principle applies here as with body types: we need the most sleep during the Kapha stage, the least during Vata time.

Maybe you're a Vata type who usually sleeps about six hours a night. But you *think* you need eight hours, so, being a Vata, you worry and worry that you're not getting enough sleep! Perhaps these numbers will reassure you.

HOW MUCH SLEEP DO YOU NEED?

Your sleep needs are largely determined by your Ayurvedic body type.

Vata = 6–7 hours

Pitta = 7–8 hours

Kapha = 8–9 hours

What Causes Insomnia?

Insomnia has two main causes, both of which we will take up in this chapter. First are a whole host of problems that all fall into the category of aggravated Vata. Vata is the organizing principle that governs movement everywhere in the body, and unbalanced Vata creates the kind of hyperactive mental activity characteristic of the inability to sleep well.

Signs of Vata aggravation include anxiety, worry, fear, and restlessness. Each of these can also *cause* disturbed Vata. Stress, excessive exercise or sexual activity for your body type, eating a too-light diet, fasting, staying up late all create agitation in the central nervous system and throw Vata out of balance. And you don't even have to have a Vata body type to have these problems.

Colleen is a 48-year-old woman who works as an administrative assistant in an insurance office. Her children are off on their own, and she has been divorced for three years. Colleen is a ruddy-faced, solidly built Pitta-Kapha type who is generally pretty easygoing. But lately problems seem to be piling up for her, and her anxiety level is high. She's got too much responsibility at the office, her youngest daughter's marriage seems to be faltering, and there are things in the house that need fixing but she doesn't know where the money's going to come from.

Night after night she lies in bed, unable to shut off her mind. First she goes over the situation at the office, thinking about how to reorganize things so she can handle it all, then fantasizing about approaching her boss and telling him one person simply can't do everything he wants done. But she's afraid to do that, because she can't afford to lose the job.

Then she goes over her daughter's situation, but in the middle of that tells herself to let go, it's not up to her anymore, she'd better think about the roof and the water heater. . . . When she does manage to fall asleep, she's so wound up that she tends to wake up again soon after with her mind in a spin. Colleen is a good example of a Pitta-Kapha constitutional type with a Vata imbalance.

The second major cause of insomnia is what we might call disturbances of routine. This can happen when you break your own regular habit patterns, such as when you cross time zones or stay up late working several nights in a row and then can't seem to get back into synch.

Joe, a 52-year-old manager of a division in a multinational corporation, frequently has to fly to Europe or Japan on business. When he was younger it was no problem, but now he finds that jet lag knocks him off his schedule so badly that he's almost always lying awake for several hours before he drifts off to sleep.

Insomnia can also be the result of being out of harmony with *nature's* regular patterns. The daily cycles on this planet of ours run through phases of Vata, Pitta, and Kapha, and we are healthiest when we organize our lives in tune with nature's rhythms. For example, going to bed during the Pitta time of night (rather than during the Kapha time) is one way insomnia can be the result of being out of synch with nature.

As we shall see, both of these causes—Vata aggravation and disturbances of routine—can easily be corrected by Ayurvedic methods.

Twenty-One Ways to Beat Insomnia

Most insomnia is caused by aggravated Vata. The problem is, sleeplessness itself increases Vata, so there can be a vicious cycle in which Vata keeps you from sleeping, and not sleeping increases Vata. Here are some proven strategies you can use to break this cycle:

1. Stick to a regular daily schedule. At least for waking up, going to bed, and meals, try to keep your schedule regular. This is one of the most powerful ways to keep Vata in balance or restore it to balance.

2. Favor the Vata-pacifying diet described in Chapter 3. Most of your food should be warm, well-cooked, and substantial. Very

light and cold foods, such as salads, are not recommended. Dairy, grains (especially wheat and rice), sweet fruits, and well-cooked vegetables are all good for balancing Vata.

3. Learn to meditate. The opposite of an agitated mind is a calm mind. Meditation allows the restless mind to settle down, producing relaxation and increased mental peace. Since meditation can have a calming effect on the mind, it is quite useful in relieving insomnia.

4. Every day do a self-massage with warm oil, as described in Chapter 4. This is very soothing and will help you avoid anxiety and stress during the day. Then you'll feel less troubled when night comes. If insomnia is really severe, you can also do this self-massage at night before getting into bed.

5. Wind down early. This is valuable for everyone, but especially if you have trouble sleeping, try to eat supper fairly early and have a peaceful, relaxing evening.

6. Avoid caffeinated drinks—coffee, tea, caffeinated cola drinks, etc.—after lunchtime. Most people are better off avoiding them altogether, as they are habit forming.

7. Watch out for medications, such as cold medicines, diet pills, etc. They often have caffeine or stronger compounds that promote insomnia. If you are taking prescribed medications and also have insomnia, read the labels or consult your physician to see if the medicines may be the culprit.

8. Avoid alcohol at night. You may think a drink or two will have a relaxing effect and help you sleep, but many studies have shown that alcohol often has the opposite effect.

9. Avoid violent or high-action television, movies, or video games, especially at night. They activate the mind too much. The same goes for loud or jarring music.

10. Eat lightly at night. Have your heaviest meal at noon. Instead of steak or pepperoni pizza at night, try some hot cereal or warm milk with toast, or rice with well-cooked vegetables. It's hard to fall asleep with a stomach full of hard-to-digest food.

11. Don't do intensive mental work just before going to bed. Try some light reading instead, or read some scriptures or uplifting literature, without any intellectual straining.

12. Listen to soothing music. Western classical and Indian classical music (*Gandharva Veda*) are good choices. You can do this before going to bed, or get in bed and listen for a while, with eyes closed, just lightly keeping your attention on the flow of the music.

13. Instead of just listening to music in the evening, sing. Singing is a wonderfully enlivening activity that increases happiness and inner peace.

14. Laughter is a powerful way to defuse stress and anxiety. Watching humorous movies or reading humorous books or comics can cheer you up and get your mind off your troubles.

15. An excellent evening activity is to spend some time playing with children.

16. Once in bed, turn off the light and lie quietly. If sleep doesn't come right away, don't read or get up. Just lie quietly. Keeping your body quietly resting will give you much of the benefit of sleep even if you don't get your full quota of sleep.

17. If you're having trouble sleeping because your mind is racing, do a mental scan of your body to see if you're having any sensations, such as a pounding heart. Putting your awareness on the sensations for a while helps take the attention away from the busy mind and has a relaxing effect.

18. Regular daily exercise often helps heal the agitation that creates insomnia. But if you have insomnia, be sure to exercise *early* in the day; late-day exercise often has just the opposite effect and keeps the body from settling down. See Chapter 7 for exercise suggestions for your body type.

19. Before getting into bed, massage your feet for a few minutes with sesame oil, ghee, or olive oil. If you have a Pitta constitution you can use coconut oil, which is cooling. This is an extremely effective way to settle the mind. Wiping the oil off with a cool cloth is said to have a calming effect on the sleep centers of the brain.

20. Drink a cup of warm milk before getting into bed. Adding a pinch of cardamom and/or nutmeg makes it more effective for inducing sleep. Adding a teaspoon of poppy seeds may also have a relaxing effect.

21. Get to bed by 10 o'clock. This will help you get into alignment with nature's rhythms, as you'll see in the next section.

Tune Your Body Clock to Nature's Rhythms for a More Restful Sleep

Another major cause of insomnia is being out of synch with nature. "Once upon a time," all over the world, people lived in harmony with Mother Nature and her rhythms. Darkness meant settling down to sleep; waking came automatically with the dawn and the singing of birds. But thanks to Thomas Edison and your local utility company, evening's dark is now just a signal to switch on the light. We can stay up as long as we want, using heating and air conditioning to be comfortable and electricity for our work or play.

However, our bodies have been deeply programmed to function in accord with nature, and they have been doing so for millions of years. One hundred years of electricity has not changed the DNA. If we go against the laws of nature operating deep within us, we may have to pay the fine.

Every day the earth passes twice through Vata, Pitta, and Kapha phases:

First Cycle	*Second Cycle*
6 A.M. to 10 A.M.= Kapha	6 P.M. to 10 P.M. = Kapha
10 A.M. to 2 P.M. = Pitta	10 P.M. to 2 A.M. = Pitta
2 P.M. to 6 P.M. = Vata	2 A.M. to 6 A.M. = Vata

According to Ayurveda, it is easiest to fall asleep and the quality of rest is deeper if we go to bed in Kapha time, before 10 P.M. Kapha has a natural property of heaviness, which will facilitate sleep. You may have noticed that around 9 P.M., at the height of Kapha time, you begin to feel sleepy. (This is particularly true of people with a Kapha body type.) Usually we fight that sleepiness, feeling that there's too much left to do. But if we went to bed early and got some deep sleep, we could do most of it much better in the morning with a fresh mind and energetic body.

Once the clock hits about 10 P.M., the Pitta cycle begins. The lively qualities of Pitta kick in, including mental alertness. You may have noticed that around that time you begin to think of all the things you need to do: balance your checkbook, write those letters, organize your desk . . . and then, as the clock approaches midnight, you've suddenly got a voracious appetite. (Also typical of Pitta time.) So you chow down, and then, finally, with a full load in your stomach for your system to work on right at the time it's geared by nature to be resting, you lie down to sleep. Good luck!

If the food won't keep you awake, Vata will. From about 2 A.M. to 6 A.M. is the Vata phase. Vata is light and airy. No wonder science has found that the last several hours of sleep in the morning are lighter, as we drift in and out between sleep, dreaming, and wakefulness. This is not the kind of sleep that will leave us refreshed in the morning.

How to Reset Your Body Clock

Are you convinced of the value of getting to bed earlier, but think it's impossible because of your long-standing habits? Don't despair—it can be done. Here is the strategy to accomplish it.

Begin by noting your usual times of going to bed and getting up and use them as a baseline. Let's say, for example, that you go to bed at 12:30 and get up at 7:30. You're a Pitta-Kapha and would ideally like to get eight hours of sleep. If you went to bed at 10:00 and got up at 6:00, you could do it.

The crucial point is your morning wake-up time. Every week, set your alarm clock to get you up 15 minutes earlier. Do this regardless of when you go to bed. Maybe you end up going to bed even later than usual on a particular night. Nevertheless, get up at 7:15. Pretty soon, your body will catch on that if it wants to get enough rest, it will have to get to sleep earlier.

Keep working back in 15-minute increments every week. You may not always find this easy. Sometimes you will have to drag yourself out of bed, and you may have trouble getting to sleep. Your daytime activity may be a little dull. But if you persevere, you will be able to reset your clock, and by being more in tune with nature's clock, you will have more energy and joy of living.

While you're doing this program, be sure to use the previous points (21 Ways to Beat Insomnia) to help you prepare for sleep. Remember to lie comfortably in bed whether sleep comes right away or not. Don't get impatient, and don't worry. It takes several weeks to establish a new habit, especially if the old one has been engrained over many years.

What if You Sleep Too Much?

Most people's sleep problems are in the "can't get enough" department. But some people sleep too much. If you find yourself wanting to sleep 9, 10, or more hours every night; if despite all that snoozing you still feel heavy and sleepy when you get up, yawn all day long, and feel like taking a nap in the afternoon, you most likely have aggravated Kapha. Kapha dosha is heavy and dull, and an excess of it in our system makes us feel slow and lazy.

The solution to excess sleep is simply to follow a Kapha-pacifying diet and daily routine. Essentially that means eating a diet that is lighter—cutting down on sweets, dairy, pasta and other wheat products, and meat—and getting more vigorous exercise.

Your diet should emphasize warm food that is as free as possible of oils, dairy, and sugar. Spicy food, such as Indian or Mexican, is good for you, but stay away from deep-fried or cheese-laden choices. Small salads are good, as the bitter taste of leafy lettuce will help curb your appetite. Start each meal with half a teaspoon of grated ginger mixed with lemon juice and a very little salt. "Just say no" to those rich, creamy desserts.

Get some vigorous exercise for at least half an hour every day during the Kapha period of the morning, between 6:00 and 10:00 A.M. See Chapter 7 for exercise recommendations for Kaphas.

Ginger tea in the morning and late afternoon is a favorite Ayurvedic recipe for combating drowsiness. *Raja's Cup*, a natural herbal mixture that tastes similar to coffee, is rejuvenating and energizing. It is available at many natural food stores.

When Your Insomnia May Need a Doctor's Care

Most insomnia can be successfully treated using the Ayurvedic methods outlined here. There are other medical reasons, however, that may need special attention.

One is known as sleep apnea, a condition usually associated with snoring and being overweight and often also with excessive alcohol consumption. People suffering with sleep apnea wake up many times during the night, often as many as 100 times, just for a moment or two before falling back to sleep. The loss of rest is severe; this condition needs to be treated by a medical specialist.

Another cause of insomnia is called myoclonis, a condition in which the person's legs jerk during sleep, awakening him or her many times.

Clinical depression also creates sleep disturbances. A person who is depressed may not feel depressed, but he or she will almost always sleep either too much or too little. Ayurvedic treatments can help a lot (see Chapter 14) but should be undertaken in conjunction with your physician, as sometimes a combined Ayurvedic and Western approach is most effective for depression.

Perhaps this children's prayer (praying before bed is often helpful for insomnia) is a fitting way to end this chapter.

Now I lay me down to sleep
I pray Thee Lord thy child to keep
Thy love guard me through the night
And wake me with the morning light.

HAPTER   13

SAY GOODBYE TO MENSTRUAL CRAMPS AND PMS

It is often said that women are closer to nature than men are. This theory certainly gains support from the fact of the monthly menstrual cycle, which links a woman so directly to the great rhythms of nature—the ebb and flow of tides, the waxing and waning of the moon, the daily cycle of the sun, the yearly cycle of seasons.

The monthly cycle represents the way women participate in the tremendous creative power of nature. As nature gives birth to countless millions and billions of species and individuals, so every woman is a partner with God and nature in the creation of life. For decades, every woman is reminded of this great capability month after month.

Despite this marvelous fact, most women experience their menstrual cycle as an inconvenience at best. At worst it is a recurring nightmare, filled with physical pain and emotional turmoil, which too easily spill over into problems in relationships. Most women—about 85 to 95 percent—experience some of the many symptoms associated with premenstrual syndrome (PMS) and 50 to 60 percent suffer from painful cramps during their period.

But this is true mostly in the modern West. Ayurvedic doctors visiting from India are often amazed at the extent of the premenstrual and menstrual problems endured by Western women. Their tradition sees the monthly cycle as a valuable opportunity for rejuvenation and purification, something that need not cause much, if any, discomfort.

In this chapter we will look at Ayurvedic secrets to help you have a smooth and comfortable experience with every phase of your monthly cycle. If you have been suffering from menstrual problems, this chapter could change your life.

Menstruation—Curse or Blessing?

Women in the Western world tend to treat their period as if it isn't happening—that is, they go to work, exercise, work around the house, entertain or attend social events, as if nothing different were going on. Many consider it a sign of weakness to even suggest that they might need to behave differently—or to be treated differently—during their period. With obligations at work and at home and a prevailing social view that isn't very understanding, women generally just take a painkiller and keep going.

The fact is, however, that something different *is* going on, and it deserves recognition and proper respect.

According to Ayurveda, a woman's monthly period serves as a time of cleansing and revitalization. If fertilization—of the egg that is released monthly—does not occur, the inner lining of the uterus (the endometrium) is sloughed off and is then removed via blood flow through the vagina. But this is not all that happens.

The body takes the opportunity given to it by the outgoing flow of blood, mucus, and tiny particles of tissue to further purify itself. All sorts of accumulated metabolic impurities (what Ayurveda calls ama) are cleared out of the body every month, rather than continue to build up to where they might be the cause of disease. This is a marvelous opportunity for cleansing, something men do not have. (Some researchers think this may be one reason women tend to live longer than men.)

If a woman *uses* this time to rest and encourage the purification process rather than continue with activity as usual, the result is rejuvenation and revitalization.

Prescription Number 1—Take It Easy

The cardinal Ayurvedic prescription for a problem-free menstrual period is, get some extra rest. Traditionally, a woman in India has been encouraged to take the first two or three days of her period, when the flow is heaviest, as a mini-vacation. Other members of her family help out with responsibilities. Of course this is easier in India, where extended families—often several generations—live together or close by. It's also easier because it's an accepted, time-honored tradition.

By contrast, as Christiane Northrup, M.D., writes in her book, *Women's Bodies, Women's Wisdom,* "This society likes action, so we often don't appreciate our need for rest and replenishment . . . time to be alone, time to rest, and time away from our daily duties." However, as Dr. Northrup suggests,

> I think that the majority of PMS cases would disappear if every modern woman retreated from her duties for three or four days each month and had her meals brought to her by someone else. (Bantam, 1994, both quotes, p. 103)

This is precisely what Ayurveda teaches. Dr. John Douillard, an expert in sports and fitness trained in Ayurvedic medicine, says, "Just as seasonal changes trigger a cascade of transitions in nature that we respond to in order to maintain balance—in terms of our dress, diet, and behavior—the monthly menstrual cycle also demands a behavioral response to the obvious physical changes taking place." That response includes getting extra rest.

But don't get the wrong idea. Resting doesn't mean staying home in bed. (Unless you have severe cramps.) It just means taking things more easy, letting yourself get more sleep at night, and reducing your activities and responsibilities as much as you can so that you don't get stressed.

For example, plan to do heavier family shopping and/or household cleaning before those days of peak flow. Try not to take on any dinner guests for those days (you don't need either the work or the anxiety of pulling it all together at this time), and keep necessary appointments to a minimum.

If you don't have a job outside your home, schedule those few days for yourself as much as you can. Catch up on reading, bill paying, organizing, and so forth. Curl up on the couch with a good book and a cup of tea (see later in the chapter for herbal tea recipes especially for women). If you have a job, see if you can take a day off. Or at least, try to make your workday shorter by not putting in overtime or long hours. If you're a student, you don't need to cut classes, but treat yourself to some time just for you. Eat lightly, especially at night, and go to bed early.

One caution: It's not recommended that you sleep during the day. This tends to build up Kapha and promotes poor circulation, heaviness, and Kapha imbalance.

In *A Woman's Best Medicine* by Nancy Lonsdorf, M.D., Veronica Butler, M.D., and Melanie Brown, Ph.D., the authors report the experiences of several women who followed these guidelines. One woman said she thought she'd "feel like a traitor to women by resting, by not working, and by not running around oblivious to my physiology throughout my period." But, she says, "now that I've experienced how it benefits my health and relationships, I've come to feel I'd be a traitor to myself if I didn't rest."

Three Different Types of Menstrual Problems—and How to Solve Them

Our old friends Vata, Pitta, and Kapha are intimately involved in the menstrual process. Kapha relates to fluids, mucus, and tissues. Blood, hormones, and the cleansing process are related to Pitta. And the flow of the menstrual fluids is governed by Vata. Any imbalance or disorder in any of these three can cause a variety of menstrual problems.

Western medicine has listed about 150 PMS symptoms and numerous symptoms of menstrual problems. As you can see in the chart on page 187, these different symptoms can be correlated with imbalances in the three doshas. Unfortunately, since this knowledge is not yet widely available, most doctors prescribe the same types of medications to all women, generally tranquilizers, muscle relaxants, pain killers, and diuretics to reduce bloating, *regardless of the person's constitutional type.* But if you can pin your symptoms down to Vata, Pitta, or Kapha it's much easier to know how to treat each unique situation and how to heal it in a completely natural way.

To bring these principles to life, let's look at two "case histories."

Charlotte, a 34-year-old physician with two young children, was plagued by years of having to put up with very uncomfortable symptoms for about five days every month. A few days prior to her period she'd become irritable (in her own words, "a vampire from

PMS and Menstrual Symptoms

VATA SYMPTOMS

Anxiety, insecurity

Insomnia

Constipation

Abdominal bloating

Lower-back pain

Painful joints

Cramps during period

Lighter flow

Dark blood

Irregular cycle

Longer-lasting periods

Mood swings

PITTA SYMPTOMS

Anger, irritability

Highly critical, argumentative

Hot flushes

Headaches (especially migraines)

Increased appetite

Excessive body heat

Burning sensations in urethra

Skin rashes

Nipples sensitive to touch

Diarrhea or loose bowels

Menstrual flow heavy and
    longer lasting

Bright-red blood

More frequent periods (shorter
    intervals between)

KAPHA SYMPTOMS

Regular cycle

Fluid retention

Breasts enlarged and tender

Tiredness, lethargy, extra sleep

Weight gain

Stiffness in back and joints

Heavy menstrual flow

Blood light-colored

Depression

Craving for sweets

Clots in blood flow

Feelings of possessiveness

Note: This chart adapted from *The Book of Ayurveda* by Judith H. Morrison and *A Woman's Best Medicine: Health, Happiness, and Long Life Through Maharishi Ayur-Veda* by Nancy Lonsdorf, M.D., Veronica Butler, M.D., and Melanie Brown, Ph.D.

hell"). When her period started the irritability decreased, but then she'd get a very heavy flow, with cramping, intense feelings of heat along with excess perspiration, and pounding migraines. Despite all this, being a doctor she felt obligated to go to work "no matter what."

Interested in natural medicine, Charlotte decided to take a doctor's training course in Maharishi Ayur-Veda. Once she learned the principles of treatment for Pitta-type menstrual problems (which was what she suffered from), she made some specific changes in her lifestyle. First, she was able to convince her partners to allow her to have a lighter schedule a couple of days every month, which she used as a "catch-up" day to get caught up on paperwork at home, as well as take things a little easier and go for walks to get some fresh air.

As soon as her PMS symptoms started, she began drinking a tea made by boiling cardamom and fennel seeds, then adding a little sugar, milk, and ghee—all very pacifying to Pitta. This greatly helped to reduce the irritability as well as the subsequent overheating and sweating. Charlotte also found that doing a coconut oil massage daily throughout the month up to her menstrual period (the full-body massage is not recommended during the actual days of menstrual flow) seemed to be effective in reducing the intensity of her PMS and menstrual symptoms. She also found an herbal formula for women, marketed as "Maharishi Ayur-Veda Women's Rasayana," to be helpful over time in reducing her symptoms. She also learned TM and felt that it helped her be more relaxed and at peace with herself throughout the day.

Here is another instance of how Ayurvedic natural remedies relieve menstrual symptoms. Laura Rose was one of those women who had trouble with her period from the time she was a teenager. It wasn't so much the cramps that troubled her, although she had them regularly enough. Rather, it was the premenstrual phase of her cycle. Predictably, several days before her period was due she would swell up. Her breasts would become enlarged and her nipples would also become very sensitive. Her appetite would increase so much she would inevitably add several pounds to her already slightly overweight frame.

But these physical symptoms were her least worry. The real problem was her emotions, which would swing out of control.

Sometimes she would find herself making critical remarks or suddenly snapping at someone. Her usual patience would seem to evaporate. Other times she became weepy and clingy. Everything looked dark and hopeless. "Life is too hard," she would say. Or, "No one really loves me." Sometimes she seemed to shift quickly from one to the other, feeling kind of "dumpy and dreary" one minute, then suddenly flaring up.

Needless to say, it was no easier for others to be around Laura Rose than it was for her to live with herself. These same patterns persisted through her twenties and early thirties, through three children and two marriages. She tried various medications, primarily for the physical symptoms, but nothing helped very much or for very long. The emotional reactions seemed to be there no matter what.

Then, at 37, she discovered Ayurveda. Her gynecologist sent her to an Ayurvedic clinic where, through an interview, a questionnaire similar to the one in this book, and a pulse diagnosis by the Ayurvedic physician she was evaluated as a Kapha-Pitta. Further questioning revealed that her usual diet was just right for creating both Kapha and Pitta imbalances.

Although she tried to eat well, her busy schedule led her to frequently indulge in cheeseburgers, fries, shakes, and other fast-food favorites. Ice cream and cookies—lots of both—would disappear when she started feeling moody. All this was exactly wrong for the Kapha aspect of her body type.

Laura Rose's other standby was Mexican food. Here the spices, cheeses, and other salty, fried, heavy choices were bad both for her Kapha and her Pitta. The result was that she built up ama during the month and aggravated her Kapha and Pitta. No wonder her moods, as well as her physical symptoms, were what they were.

Laura Rose's situation was a bit complex. If the doctor prescribed too many heating remedies (spicy foods, ginger tea, etc.), that would tend to reduce Kapha, but at the expense of making Laura's Pitta flare up in irritation and outbursts of anger. If the wrong cooling recommendations were given (such as ice cream, which can be very soothing and balancing to Pittas) that would likely aggravate her Kapha.

The doctor prescribed five key strategies for Laura Rose to follow:

1. Sip *small* amounts of hot water regularly during the day (this would help clear out ama without aggravating Pitta dosha).

2. Do half an hour of aerobic exercise every day except during her period, when she was told to walk half an hour.

3. Lean toward the Kapha-balancing diet, emphasizing warm, light foods, with some whole grains and a lot of fresh vegetables, and eliminating or greatly minimizing red meat, all dairy products except skim milk, all products with refined sugar (including cookies, ice cream, candies, sodas, etc.), and cutting down on wheat-based foods such as pasta and bread.

4. Also watch out for too much Pitta-increasing foods, foods that are salty, spicy, or sour.

5. Eat her main meal for lunch, and have a light, early supper.

Just following these for one month made a huge difference, greatly reducing her PMS symptoms. Within six months on this program, Laura Rose had hardly any symptoms at all.

You can gain the same benefits in your own life, whether your symptoms are as dramatic as Laura Rose's or you have just some minor discomfort. The key is to check any symptoms you might have against the preceding chart to gain a deeper understanding of what is causing them. Then use the knowledge you've gained throughout this book to help you prevent and heal those symptoms.

For example, if your symptoms are primarily in the Vata-related list, be sure to favor the Vata-pacifying diet, Vata-balancing exercises, and take herbs or herb teas for reducing Vata. The same for Pitta and Kapha. You will be amazed at the results.

Ten Ayurvedic Secrets for Easier Periods

Now that we've considered specific symptoms caused by imbalances in Vata, Pitta, and Kapha, here are some effective strategies any woman can use to minimize or eliminate problems at all phases of the menstrual cycle. Use these tips during the time of your menstrual flow, particularly during the heaviest two or three days at the beginning.

1. *Get plenty of rest.* As we've already talked about, the most important thing you can do during your period is to cut back on your activity and get extra rest, especially during your days of peak flow. This will not only be healing for you, it will also provide a basis for more energy and happiness during the rest of the month and for better health far into the future.

2. *Favor your inward tendencies.* You may have noticed a natural tendency to turn inward during these days, to want to be quiet and settled, even protected from the usual hustle and bustle of life. Try to arrange your schedule so you can have that peace and quiet for a few days. You deserve it! Favor that part of you that's more introspective, not constantly outgoing and active.

Remember: It's not selfish to take care of yourself. Caring for your health is not self-indulgent, it's smart. It's the first step toward taking the best care of others and of all your responsibilities.

3. *Minimize exercise.* Some medical authorities now recommend vigorous exercise to women during their periods, but this is not the Ayurvedic prescription. Exercise during the rest of the month is highly recommended, but during your period, take it easy. Skip your dance class and don't do aerobic exercise or even perform the yoga postures in Chapter 7.

All the exercise you need for these few days is just a 15- to 30-minute walk. A key reason: Vata is dominating your physiology during your menstrual flow, and the best type of exercise for balancing Vata is gentle, smooth, and steady. Walking is ideal. Even if you're a competitive athlete, I recommend that you cut way back on your training regime during these few days.

4. *Eat light.* Warm, lighter foods like soups and steamed vegetables are best during your period. You might even want to try a purely liquid diet on Day 1 (such as soups, herbal teas, fresh juices, plain warm water). In general, favor the Vata-balancing diet for these few days, but beware of heavier foods that are ama producing, such as cheese, yogurt, and red meat. You'll feel better if you cut back on fried, salty, and highly spiced foods, too. Following these recommendations should help reduce cramping as well as bloating.

5. *Opt for quick showers.* Although you might find a hot bath soothing, particularly if you tend to have cramps, Ayurveda recom-

HERBS TO HELP WITH YOUR PERIOD

Numerous herbs and herbal teas can be helpful in regulating the menstrual cycle; they are soothing and help relieve cramps and promote a comfortable flow. Here are several:

- Raspberry-leaf tea.
- Hibiscus flowers. These make a delicious tea hot or cold. Raspberry and hibiscus can be combined.
- Ginger tea.
- Mugwort (tea or capsules) helps regulate the cycle and relieve cramping.
- *Dong Quai* (also known as Angelica). "Perhaps the best herb for regulating the menstrual cycle," according to Dr. Vasant Lad and David Frawley, authors of *The Yoga of Herbs*. Remember that if you use honey to sweeten any teas, use raw, uncooked honey and wait until the tea has cooled down enough to sip comfortably before adding the honey.

mends that bathing be limited to quick showers (on the cooler side) or even just sponging down. Bathing in hot water will tend to increase the flow.

6. *Postpone sex.* The traditional texts of Ayurveda recommend refraining from sex—not just intercourse, but all sexual activity—during the days of the period. As the authors of *A Woman's Best Medicine* point out, "This recommendation is not based either on the desirability of a woman at this time or on a woman's desires; it is based on a sound principle for health." Sexual activity at this time, they say, will tend to create Vata imbalance.

7. *Steer clear of tampons.* Although the ancient Ayurvedic texts have nothing to say about this modern invention, the doctors who wrote *A Woman's Best Medicine* recommend that you use external absorbent pads instead of tampons whenever possible or convenient, especially at night or when you are home. The tampons tend to restrict the blood flow, which can disturb Vata, leading to cramps and other symptoms of Vata aggravation.

8. *Rx for cramps.* If you have strong cramps, Dr. Vasant Lad, director of the Ayurvedic Institute in Albuquerque, New Mexico, recommends a tablespoon of aloe vera gel with two pinches of black pepper "three times a day until cramps disappear."

9. *Sip hot water.* Even if you can't bathe in hot water (see number 5), you *can* drink it. During the days of your period take a few sips of hot water every half hour to an hour. This is balancing to Vata, eliminates ama, and will help prevent cramps.

10. *Pacify Vata with warmth.* Cramps generally respond to warmth. If you are hurting, you can use some warm sesame oil to *gently* massage your abdomen and lower back. Follow with a hot-water bottle, either in front or back, as you wish.

Five Master Keys to Make Your Whole Cycle Comfortable

The previous tips were specifically for the time of your menstrual flow. The following will help if you use them throughout the month on a regular basis.

1. *Get regular exercise.* One of the most important ways you can help ensure comfortable periods and an absence of premenstrual symptoms is to get regular exercise. Chapter 7 is filled with exercise recommendations for your body type, and I won't repeat them here, except to say that I especially recommend the Sun Salutation and Yoga postures. The stretching and bending are highly beneficial for massaging the internal organs and eliminating ama. Note that the cobra and locust postures are specifically known for their benefits to the female reproductive system.

2. *Watch your diet.* One of the main sources of both PMS symptoms and menstrual cramps is the buildup of the metabolic impurities known as ama. Menstruation can be viewed as your body's monthly toxic-cleanup program, but don't take unfair advantage of it by packing your body with gunk that will have to be eliminated. The more ama that needs to be cleared out, the more difficulty you are likely to have with PMS and menstrual discomfort. So avoid junk food (salt, fats and fried foods, refined sugar, white flour), minimize caffeine and alcohol consumption, eliminate heavy and hard-to-digest red meat, minimize Kapha- and ama-producing dairy foods such as yogurt, ice cream, and hard cheeses.

Follow the diet plan for your body type (see Chapter 3). Sip hot water regularly throughout the day. If you do these things conscientiously, you should find a significant decrease in any PMS or menstrual difficulties that have been plaguing you.

3. *Get regular rest.* Once again I want to emphasize rest, but this time, the importance of sleeping in a regular rhythm. As we've discussed in Chapter 6, Ayurveda strongly recommends following a regular routine. One of the central pillars of your routine is your bedtime, which should be early, as close to 10 P.M. as you can make it. Both going to bed late and erratic lifestyle habits with varying bedtimes and mealtimes aggravate Vata and set the stage for Vata-related symptoms such as cramps, bloating, mood swings, and so forth.

4. *Daily oil massage.* Your daily *abhyanga* or oil massage (see Chapter 4) will help pacify Vata and keep you in balance. It will also reduce stress and help you sleep well.

5. *Meditate.* Another powerful stress reducer is meditation. "Women who practice meditation or other methods of deep relaxation are able to alleviate many of their PMS symptoms," says Dr. Christiane Northrup. "Any modality that decreases stress can help menstrual period regulation because of the profound link between emotional or psychological stress and biochemical imbalance," she says. Ayurveda could not agree more strongly. Regular meditation helps to lower anxiety and tension and create balance in the physiology.

These helpful secrets from the timeless wisdom of Ayurveda can help you toward appreciating your connection to nature's constant rhythms and flows. If you follow the guidelines in this chapter, you may find that PMS and other menstrual problems quickly become a distant memory.

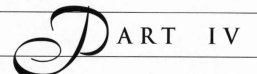

UNFOLD YOUR FULL POTENTIAL

THE AYURVEDIC WAY TO MENTAL AND EMOTIONAL WELLNESS

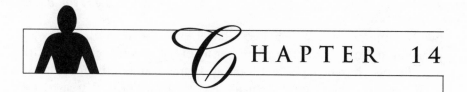

BEAT THE BLUES
AYURVEDIC SECRETS TO HELP YOU OVERCOME DEPRESSION

If it sometimes seems that you and others around you are feeling blue, you may be right: During any six-month period at least nine million American adults are suffering from depression.

According to the National Institute of Mental Health, more than 20 million Americans suffer a "medically significant" episode of depression at least once in their lifetime. Countless millions of others suffer from minor periods of sadness, low energy, and lack of motivation. Just about everyone has the blues sometimes, whether caused by external circumstances, internal conflicts and indecisions, hormones, or by being tired and overwhelmed.

Although Western psychiatry has made some progress toward reducing the symptoms of depression, treatment remains largely unsatisfactory. Most medications for major depression have strong side effects, and there really is no effective treatment for people who are just feeling temporarily low. Very importantly, Western medicine knows no way to prevent depression, so at least half the people treated for it suffer recurrences.

By contrast, Ayurvedic methods of treating depression are gentle, natural, and effective. They contribute to a long-lasting state of balance that may reduce the tendency toward recurrences.

The Ayurvedic perspective on depression brings a fresh wave of hope for millions of men and women. It offers a more complete understanding of the nature and causes of depression; more effec-

197

tive treatment without negative side effects; the real possibility of prevention; and promotion of higher levels of psychological health.

In this chapter we'll first look at depression as it is understood in Western medicine and then as it is understood and treated by Ayurveda. If depression is a concern of yours, I believe that this chapter will offer a light at the end of the tunnel—a genuine hope that you or someone you care about will be able to enjoy life fully again.

That's because Ayurvedic methods not only increase balance in the body, they also progressively raise the overall level of inner contentment, which naturally works to prevent depression. What better vaccine against depression could there be than happiness?

The Western Perspective on Depression

When you are depressed, life loses its charm. Nothing matters. Nothing seems to be working out. Energy is low, decisions are difficult to make, and even simple everyday tasks feel overwhelming. Everything looks flat, bleak, and gray, and you feel certain it has always been and always will be the same way. You tend to focus only on the negative side of things, seeing the worst in yourself, your life, your friends, your accomplishments, your prospects. Self-esteem hits rock bottom.

Symptoms of Depression

The symptoms of depression include

- Persistent sad or "empty" mood
- Loss of interest in friends and usual activities
- Insomnia, early morning awakening, or oversleeping
- Anxiety, irritability, restlessness
- Low energy, fatigue, "can't get going"
- Poor appetite and weight loss, or sometimes the reverse: overeating and weight gain
- Difficulty concentrating and making decisions
- Decreased sex drive
- Feelings of worthlessness and guilt

- Feelings of hopelessness and helplessness
- Frequent crying spells
- Suicidal thoughts

In a milder depression, you either have fewer symptoms, or the symptoms feel less intense. In a more severe depression, the number and intensity of symptoms is greater.

Causes of Depression

There are three basic causes of depression. The first is external. A high degree of stress, such as the death of someone close to you, serious financial problems, or a prolonged stressful situation that seems inescapable or unresolvable (a bad marriage, a tyrannical parent, a child repeatedly in trouble, etc.), can produce a depression. This often takes the form of hopelessness: There seems to be "no way out."

The second factor is biological. A genetic predisposition to depression is apparently passed on from generation to generation, just as the tendency to develop a physical illness such as diabetes is passed on. That seems to be why some people without unusual outer difficulties develop the condition, often in their late twenties or early thirties (although depression can appear at any time, from childhood to old age).

The third causative factor is "psychological." Freud said that depression is "anger turned inward." That means that if a person is frustrated and angry long enough without expressing it, he (or she) may turn the anger and hatred inward, against himself (or herself) and end up depressed.

Whatever the cause of depression, a biological imbalance always accompanies it, and both Western medicine and Ayurveda direct their treatment toward correcting this imbalance, but in different ways.

Types of Depression

Although the subjective experience of depression is fairly universal, Western medicine has defined three major types:

1. *Adjustment reaction* lasts weeks to months and usually follows some specific stressful event in one's life, such as a divorce, the loss of a job, or the death of a loved one. With time, a person usually recovers spontaneously. Talk therapy to facilitate understanding or to release pent-up feelings, or the temporary use of anti-depressant medication to relieve the symptoms, may accelerate the healing.

2. *Dysthymic disorder* is a chronic form of depression with moderate symptoms that may linger on for a long time, even for years. People suffering from this kind of depression live in an emotional desert; as the months of depression drag on, they take little pleasure in life, operate on low energy, and feel truly hopeless about their future.

3. *Major depression* has symptoms that are more severe, including dark moods, sleep disturbances, appetite disturbances, feelings of hopelessness, and even suicidal thoughts. Major depression is usually preceded by a prolonged period of stress, but the genetic factor is frequently involved also.

Standard Treatments of Depression and Their Shortcomings

The first type of depression frequently heals spontaneously. Both the first and second may respond to talk therapy. But talk therapy is rarely sufficient to treat major depression. Because there is some biochemical imbalance in the brain that must be addressed, other treatments are required.

The two biological treatments that are mainstays of Western psychiatric treatment for major depression are

1. electro-convulsive therapy (ECT), commonly known as "shock treatment" and
2. anti-depressant medications. These strong medications usually act upon either of two neurotransmitters in the brain, norepinephrine or serotonin, which are in low supply in depressed individuals.

People who use these medications frequently suffer significant side effects such as dry mouth, tachycardia (rapid heart rate), constipation, dizziness, sexual dysfunction, jitteriness, blurred vision, and memory impairment. The memory loss stemming from ECT is often so severe that memory of the entire period surrounding the shock treatment is completely wiped out.

Even when the medications successfully alleviate symptoms in the short run—which they frequently do accomplish—*at least 50 percent of major depressions recur.* In other words, the medications developed by Western medicine are effective for temporary relief of symptoms, but a long-range program to maintain mental and physical balance and prevent recurrences is unknown.

This has led some physicians to advocate that people who have once been treated for major depression remain on anti-depressant medications all the time as a preventive measure, even though they may have to suffer from the side effects all the time. Significant numbers of people with depressions ranging from mild to severe are taking anti-depressant medications on a daily basis.

These treatments *at best* help people regain their baseline level of functioning prior to their struggle with depression. The concept of helping the person grow toward levels of happiness *higher* than the baseline level is simply not an option with current methods of treatment.

Also, as mentioned, no meaningful help is available for the tens of millions of normal, healthy people who experience a minor depression from time to time in their lives. These less severe depressions have little status in the field of psychiatry. Because they are not serious enough to be classified as "critical," nothing is done about them. And yet such depressions can be very disabling. Insomnia, irritability, sluggishness, and so forth, adversely affect one's work and one's personal life.

If a person knows he or she is prone to falling into depression, can anything be done to prevent it from happening? The unfortunate truth is that modern medicine is still in its infancy in this regard. In recent years, humanistic psychologists and others have realized that healthful lifestyles can have a positive effect upon mental health in general, and some interest is growing in applying the principles of preventive medicine to mental health; but it is just a bare beginning.

Restoring Balance: Ayurvedic Body-Type Treatments for Depression

From the standpoint of Ayurveda there are two main causes of depression. The first is lack of awareness of one's deeper, inner Self. The second is an imbalance in the three doshas, Vata, Pitta, and Kapha. Let's look at this one first.

From your study of Ayurveda so far, you might think that depression is primarily born of excess Kapha dosha, since the Kapha qualities of heaviness, dullness, and slowness resemble some of the symptoms of depression. This would be a good guess. However, classical Ayurvedic texts clearly describe three different types of depression, along with their origin and treatment. These texts—and clinical experience—show that depression can result not only from Kapha imbalance, but from aggravated Vata or Pitta as well.

How to Treat a Vata-Type Depression

One October afternoon, Bill consulted Dr. Browning, a physician trained in Ayurvedic medicine, complaining of depression. He said that he felt tired all the time, so tired that he could barely get through the day at work. Once he got home, he couldn't muster up the motivation to do anything more than watch TV. Even weekends, on which he used to love to go bicycling or hiking with friends, had turned into a lethargic round of TV, dozing, and sitting

HOW TO HEAL A VATA-TYPE DEPRESSION

How to Tell if Your Depression Is Due to Vata Imbalance
In addition to your subjective feelings of depression or low mood and energy:

- Vata pulse
- skin cold to the touch; you will feel cold, may even experience shivering
- poor appetite, weight loss
- digestive problems, constipation
- super-sensitive
- anxious
- can't sleep
- excessive talking about nothing and everything
- fearful
- restless, can't sit still
- frequent urination
- usually Vata constitution and appearance: thin body, small eyes, dry skin, cracking joints, etc.

Factors That Contribute to Vata Depression

- too much sex or frequent masturbation
- overactivity
- exposure to cold or wind
- autumn or winter season
- overexercising
- irregular hours
- staying up late

Treatment of Vata Depression

- Follow Vata-pacifying diet (see Chapter 3). Favor foods that are strengthening, heavier, warm. Avoid salads, fruits; favor whole grains, vegetables cooked in oil and spiced, dairy products, nuts.
- Maintain a regular daily routine with early bedtime.
- Daily abhyanga (oil massage).
- Keep warm; take warm baths or showers.
- Mild exercise such as walking or yoga postures.
- Daily meditation.
- Listen to relaxing music such as classical or Indian classical (Gandharva Veda).
- Use Vata-balancing herbs such as anise, cinnamon, cumin, ginger, gotu kola, licorice, nutmeg, sesame seeds, and valerian (for sleep).

---

around the house alone. At night he had trouble falling asleep and then woke up several times.

Bill was tall and thin and appeared nervous and restless; he was having trouble sitting still. Just from these observations, Dr. Browning easily guessed that his complaint originated in excess Vata.

From the pulse diagnosis, he determined that Bill did have a predominantly Vata constitution and that there was an aggravation of Vata dosha in his system. Dr. Browning then asked Bill a number of questions to determine what it was in his life circumstances or routine that had created the unbalanced condition.

He found quite a number of things. First, Bill was prone to staying up late and to keeping erratic hours. Both of these aggravate Vata. He also drank quite a bit of coffee, and his diet included a lot of salads. Caffeine is very aggravating to Vata, which is speedy enough as it is, and salads are also not the best for this already light, airy, and cold constitutional type. In addition, it was autumn, a time when winds and cooling weather frequently aggravate Vata. Bill also tended to exercise heavily and had probably worn himself out on those hiking trips.

Dr. Browning gave Bill a number of recommendations to bring Vata back into balance. First, he urged him to get onto a more structured routine, with an earlier bedtime. He told him to wean himself gradually from caffeine and to add more warm and "heavier" foods to his diet (such as soups, pasta, rice with well-cooked vegetables), to help pacify the excess Vata. He also suggested that he wear a hat when out in the autumn wind (even if the temperature was not very cold) and recommended the set of yoga postures in Chapter 7. The doctor told Bill that hiking was fine, so long as he didn't overdo it.

He suggested meditation, which would help to settle him without threatening his dynamism. He also recommended a daily oil massage, either to the whole body, time permitting, or at least to the head and the soles of his feet. Dr. Browning recommended some herbs that were quite inexpensive and would have no negative side effects. These could be taken as a tea—warm drinks are soothing to Vata—or in capsules. These changes in lifestyle, if Bill followed them, would begin to alleviate the depression within a few days.

As mentioned, one problem with Vata personality types is that they have difficulty doing anything at all in a consistent way. Even when they are convinced something, such as an exercise program, is good for them, they will frequently do it only sporadically. This is especially true when Vata is out of balance, and the resulting erratic lifestyle will tend to maintain or increase the imbalance. It is thus very helpful for Vatas to do their best to develop consistency.

Although it took a couple of meetings with Bill to convince him of this, after that he was able to adhere reasonably well to his new program, and within a short time he was feeling significantly better.

How to Treat a Pitta-Type Depression

Now let's look at an example of a Pitta depression. One afternoon an attractive red-headed woman named Ellen went to a psychotherapist trained in Ayurvedic natural medicine. Ellen was about 30, of medium height and build, with a few freckles, and an intense

HOW TO HEAL A PITTA-TYPE DEPRESSION

How to Tell if Your Depression Is Due to Pitta Imbalance
In addition to your subjective feelings of depression and low energy or dark mood:

- Pitta pulse
- Pitta appearance and constitution: medium to strong build, often red or light hair, fair complexion, freckles
- feel hot and be sensitive to heat
- skin reddish and may feel hot to the touch
- desire to eat sweets a lot, and butter, ghee, or creamy desserts
- irritable and easily angered
- hair falling out or turning white
- ulcers or feeling of heat in stomach
- diarrhea
- redness in eyes

Factors That Contribute to Pitta Depression
- frequently occurs in summer months
- not wearing hat in the sun
- taking hot showers
- not covering head with cool cloth in steam or sauna
- eating hot foods (both temperature and spice)
- missing meals, especially lunch
- frequent experience of anger or irritation

Treatment of Pitta Depression
- Follow Pitta-pacifying diet (see Chapter 3). In general avoid hot and spicy foods, red meat, fish, vinegar, cheese, alcohol, and tobacco. Favor cool (not ice cold) drinks, a vegetarian diet, dairy products (not yogurt), sweet fruit, most vegetables and grains.
- Stay out of the sun; keep cool.
- Minimize hot baths or showers.
- Moderate exercise such as swimming, bicycling.
- Take largest meal at noon; don't skip lunch.
- Panchakarma purification procedures.
- Daily meditation.
- Listen to relaxing music such as classical or Indian classical (*Gandharva Veda*).

(Box text continues on page 206)

- Use Pitta-reducing herbs such as aloe, burdock, chrysanthemum, co-conut, coriander, cumin, mint, pomegranate, sandalwood, shatavari (Indian asparagus), and natural sugar.
- Daily coconut oil massage

---

gaze. She was impatient, apparently because the therapist had kept her waiting a few minutes; she mentioned that she hoped the session would not go overtime and force her to be late for her racquetball match.

When Ellen said she was depressed and the therapist asked her to talk more about it, she revealed that she had aspirations for a position in her company that had recently been given to somebody else. She felt that she was much more qualified than the man who got the job and that he got it primarily because he was a man. "I'm smarter, more productive, and more successful than he is," she said, making a fist as she spoke.

On closer investigation, however, underneath the rage was a feeling of failure. "I've been working hard for this position, and I didn't get it. What will happen now? Will I ever really succeed?"

Her pulse revealed that Ellen was a predominantly Pitta personality type, suffering from aggravated Pitta. Pitta people set high standards, can be very competitive, and tend to be perfectionistic. They are virtually addicted to success and are always checking to see how they measure up to their own high standards. Any failure, real or imagined, is likely to cause a depression.

As the therapist questioned Ellen about her lifestyle and routine, he found that she was fond of sunbathing and outdoor sports and went for lunch several times a week to a Mexican restaurant where she ate hot, spicy foods. For a person of Pitta constitution, getting too much exposure to sun and heat or eating too many spicy foods are more than sufficient to aggravate Pitta. When these factors were combined with the perceived rejection and failure at work, Ellen's Pitta became severely aggravated. Ellen didn't smoke or drink much alcohol, but if a Pitta person uses these substances for a calming effect, this would further aggravate Pitta.

Ellen had chosen this particular therapist because she was adamant that she did not want to take antidepressant drugs. She wasn't excited about eliminating the Mexican foods, however, or about staying out of the sun, but she said she'd try it for a month, along with the Pitta-pacifying diet the therapist laid out for her.

The counselor told her that for Pittas, perhaps the most important factor to maintain balance was to take life a little easier. Imbalanced Pitta always wants to compete, to strive, to push ahead, but that very pushing further aggravates Pitta dosha. She needed to relax and to "lighten up." He suggested that Ellen learn meditation to help her relax and also that she create more leisure time in her schedule to laugh more and enjoy lighter entertainment. Because Pitta individuals tend, deep down, to feel alone in the world, the company of friends often has a balancing influence.

Although she was skeptical (another Pitta characteristic), Ellen applied her highly developed self-discipline to the regimen set for her. In addition, she went for therapy twice a week. Within a couple of months her depression had significantly lifted and she ended her therapy, seeing the value of her Pitta-balancing routine and vowing to stick with it.

How to Treat a Kapha-Type Depression

Kapha depression often occurs in the colder months or in early springtime, due to the increase of cold or moisture, which are both Kapha-aggravating factors. Eating rich foods or a large quantity of oily, salty, sweet, sour, or cold foods also increases the risk. Excessive sleep (particularly in the daytime) is another risk factor for aggravating Kapha.

Overeating, not properly chewing food, or reading or watching television while eating produce *ama,* a metabolic impurity in the system particularly associated with excess Kapha. Improperly digested food results in inadequately metabolized food, which accumulates in the body and interferes with normal cellular functions. This accumulated ama—said to be a heavy, sticky substance—tends to block the channels of the body, such as the blood and lymphatic systems.

The biochemical properties of red meat also increase the tendencies toward Kapha-type depression. They are heavy and have a dulling effect on mind and body.

These factors cause an accumulation in the body of the Kapha metabolic impurities, which are sticky, cold, and heavy. This accumulation then brings on the symptoms that characterize Kapha depression.

The ancient Ayurvedic physicians also noted that decreased exposure to sunlight is a factor that can contribute to Kapha depres-

HOW TO HEAL A KAPHA-TYPE DEPRESSION

How to Tell if Your Depression Is Due to Kapha Imbalance

In addition to your subjective feelings of depression and low energy or dark mood:

- Kapha pulse
- feeling cold
- overeating
- tendency to occur in winter or spring months
- usually a Kapha body type
- low energy
- paleness of skin
- overweight
- oversleeping
- loss of ability to experience pleasure

Factors That Contribute to Kapha Depression

- tendency toward inactivity and lack of exercise, laziness
- eating heavy diet
- not dressing properly for the cold weather
- eating cold instead of warm foods
- increase of ama due to eating wrong foods, or to poor eating habits such as not chewing food sufficiently, reading or watching TV while eating, etc.
- daytime sleep

Treatment of Kapha Depression

- Follow Kapha-pacifying diet, especially spicy, hot foods, light soups (see Chapter 3). Favor apples and pears, grains such as barley, buckwheat, millet, and corn. Honey is the only sweetener good for Kapha. All spices (except salt) are good. Minimize oils and fats, wheat and rice, cold food in general, sweets, nuts, rich desserts, red meat, most dairy.
- Use heating herbs such as ginger, pepper, turmeric. Drink ginger tea.
- Get vigorous exercise such as jogging, bicycling, aerobics.
- Walk or exercise in the sun, but don't get too much exposure on skin.
- Panchakarma purification procedure.
- Daily practice of meditation.
- Avoid daytime sleep.

sion. This is why many people tend toward depression in the darker winter months. Walking outside in the sun for a few minutes a day is emphasized in Ayurveda as one of the best ways to prevent mental illness, especially depression.

Western psychiatry has recently pinpointed a type of depression known as seasonal affective disorder (SAD), which occurs during the darker months of the year. SAD is characterized by oversleeping, overeating, apathetic mood, feelings of "hard to get going," loss of ambition and drive, and weight gain, all symptoms of Kapha depression.

Several years ago, when some researchers suggested that people with SAD could be treated with light, a controversy erupted in the mental health profession. Most doctors, accustomed to treating depression with powerful drugs, were vehemently opposed to the idea that something as natural and simple as light could be used instead. Yet, light treatment has proven to be highly effective.

Of course, absence of light is only one factor in an entire syndrome. SAD, with all the symptoms of a Kapha depression, occurs in cold, moist, heavy winter weather because when Kapha increases in the environment, it also tends to increase inside us. Thus, for a person with Kapha-induced depression, the cure is a Kapha-reducing regimen. Specific herbs that reduce Kapha, such as ginger and pepper, foods that are spicy, hot, and dry, and hot liquids such as teas and light soups are valuable. More vigorous exercise is called for, as is some exposure to sunlight or, if the weather is bad, high-intensity artificial light as mentioned earlier.

Important note: Depression can be just a temporary heavy mood or a long-lasting and serious mental illness. If you are feeling low, try the Ayurvedic remedies I have just described. However, if the depression lingers consult a physician or mental health professional. You can continue with these self-treatments, which will help you regain balance and maintain it in the long run. But you may need some additional measures to help you cope with the immediate situation.

If you go to a doctor and wish to continue with the Ayurvedic recommendations, you might mention that Western antidepressant medications typically require a minimum of three weeks to take effect, but Ayurvedic treatments, though gentler, begin to produce results more quickly, within a few days or even a few hours. The two are completely compatible. Mental health professionals have found that when people begin to experience improvement from the

Ayurvedic treatments, they frequently desire to discontinue the stronger antidepressant drugs as quickly as possible, in order to avoid any continued side effects. Ask your doctor to monitor the situation with you.

Heal Depression by Shining Your Inner Light

Now let's explore another aspect of depression. This may seem more abstract than what we've been talking about, but it is important, ground-breaking knowledge for mental health in general and depression in particular. So bear with me if these next pages aren't filled with specific remedies: this is about one very important method that we could almost call a super-remedy.

In Ayurveda, the Self, one's inmost spiritual center, is said to be a field of contentment and joy. (The term that is often used is "bliss consciousness.") When our attention is directed exclusively outward to the objects of experience and we don't meditate or have deep experiences of prayer or other spiritual practices, we easily lose touch with the unbounded awareness and bliss of the Self. This outward turning of awareness is known in Maharishi Ayur-Veda as "object referral"; turning inward to gain the experience of the Self is called "Self-referral."

Self-referral is an *experience*, not an intellectual exercise or a type of introspection. A depressed person who looks within will typically find nothing but dark and hopeless thoughts and feelings; this is not what I mean. I'm talking about a direct inner perception of the pure consciousness underlying all our thoughts and feelings, an inner quietness or silence, a state of pure awareness or pure being that is blissful and expansive in nature.

This experience is so important because ultimately all happiness comes from within. This statement may seem extreme. "What about my wife or husband, what about the beauty of nature, what about my children? I derive great happiness from them," you might argue. But the truth of this principle is immediately apparent if you just think about the topic of discussion in this chapter. A depressed person is not able to derive happiness from anything, even things and people that formerly gave great joy.

That is the great frustration of anyone trying to help a depressed person. Whatever you try to bring to them or remind them of, the person is as if inwardly wearing dark glasses and hence sees nothing but darkness everywhere.

We all verify this principle ourselves, every day. As our inner moods shift, our ability to enjoy the world around us shifts correspondingly. In a happy mood, we can derive joy from the smallest, most insignificant-seeming things. In a dark mood, everything is a drag.

Depression is an extreme form of object-referral, in which you completely lose touch with the inner happiness of the Self. It is as if the doors of the bank are locked and you are doomed to eternal poverty.

But any unhappiness, not just depression, has the same cause. The more you lose touch with the joy and freedom of the Self, the more you are bound to feel frustrated and unhappy. As you gain readmittance into the inner dimension of fullness, unhappiness disappears.

Another way to phrase this is, to treat unhappiness, increase happiness. To treat darkness, increase light. This is a simple but profoundly effective way of treating depression. Here is a dramatic example.

Healing Depression with Self-Referral: A Case History

Mary said she was a "wreck" when she finally forced herself to seek help. A successful attorney with a good job, she had endured severe depression for months before she made an appointment with a psychiatrist. Her persistent feelings of darkness and despair had become unbearable.

"My life and my future seem empty," she said to the doctor; "I can barely force myself to go to work, even though I know I have to—I have three children to support.

"I seem to have totally lost my appetite," she added, "and I've lost almost 15 pounds. I toss and turn for hours before I fall asleep, and I can't seem to make up my mind about anything." She also reported frequent crying spells and a great deal of difficulty concentrating and functioning at work.

Frightening memories from childhood prompted Mary to try to harm herself, first by cutting herself with a knife, then by trying to drive off a bridge. Because she couldn't be left alone with such powerful feelings, she had to be hospitalized in a locked psychiatric unit, with 24-hour-a-day supervision. More intensive psychotherapy was done with her in the hospital, but this only intensified the suicidal thoughts and the severity of the depression.

In a case as severe as Mary's, Western psychiatry currently has two alternatives: shock treatment or antidepressant medication. She refused shock treatment. Several medications were tried, but because she was very sensitive to them and experienced side effects, she couldn't take doses high enough to help.

The doctor thought this would be an appropriate time to discuss alternative forms of treatment with Mary. He told her that according to Ayurveda, a central reason for her depression was lack of contact with a deep aspect of herself that was a field of happiness and fullness. She was very receptive. Despite her depressed state, she was able to appreciate that opening up to that part of herself might be precisely what she needed to heal her life.

She felt particularly drawn toward meditation. Because she was so disgusted with the side effects of the medicines she had taken, a natural approach, which she could utilize by herself and which would be easy and comfortable to perform, seemed like a wonderful and welcome change.

She was taught the Transcendental Meditation technique. Immediately she enjoyed a deep experience of pure consciousness, a very quiet, peaceful level of awareness, and reported that she felt "filled with light and happiness." Her meditation experiences left her with such an intense degree of inner fullness that she herself was startled by the transformation—as were the nurses and other mental health professionals on the unit.

Within a few days—literally—most of her symptoms were gone. Her appearance was almost immediately brighter, and everyone could see that her mood was significantly improved. "My appetite is back," she said, "and I can concentrate better." Most important, she felt a strong desire to live. She saw many wonderful possibilities for her life in the future and was hopeful. From darkness and suicidal despair, her outlook had become positive and hopeful.

The magnitude and rapidity of the changes in Mary surprised even the doctor. He wondered if the sudden transformation might be due to what is known as the "placebo effect." Did the expectation that she would be helped trigger a temporary improvement? He kept her in the hospital for another few days to be sure. But the changes were genuine and lasting; she continued to improve day by day.

Mary's transformation was even measured biochemically, using the *dexamethasone suppression test*, which at the time was a standard way to determine the degree of depression in a patient. The normal range in a nondepressed person is a natural cortisone level under 5. Before learning meditation, Mary had measured as high as 41. Three weeks after learning meditation and being released from the hospital, her level had dropped to 7.

With continuing regular meditation combined with therapy, Mary made rapid progress. A year later she was functioning well at work and continuing to feel better. The depression had not returned. She appeared to be a different person, much more self-reliant, more trusting of others, and deeply appreciative of her meditation and the contribution it was making to her life.

Restoring Self-Referral

If this story sounds exaggerated (it is accurate except for a name change), consider something that *might* have happened to Mary. When she finally sought help, she felt hopeless and trapped and perceived herself, as she said, "getting older, with no hope for happiness anywhere on the horizon." Her marriage had fallen apart and she was lonely, struggling to maintain a good life for herself and her children.

Now suppose that, by chance, she met a warm, loving, and responsible man, fell in love, and was loved in return. How would she feel? Her inner world would suddenly be so much brighter. The weight of hopelessness would fall away. Imagine the sense of joy and freedom she would feel, the almost intoxicating release from restricting boundaries. Now anything would seem possible.

But—it would all be dependent upon the change in her outer circumstances. And that could change again, in any direction.

The sense of freedom and blossoming possibilities gained from the experience of the inner Self is analogous to our hypothetical romance, with one added advantage: It is entirely one's own. It is not dependent upon a new romance or a new job; you don't have to rely on a change of outer circumstances. Inner happiness and joy bubble up spontaneously, so depression begins to dissolve. Life and progress again feel possible and desirable.

If meditation could turn around a depression as serious as Mary's, it can certainly shine light into the far less severe blue moods we all go through. That is why I always recommend meditation to anyone with depression, and indeed to everyone who wants to expand his or her boundaries and grow into a better life.

"DON'T WORRY, BE HAPPY"— AYURVEDIC SECRETS FOR OVERCOMING ANXIETY

If you're a human being in the late twentieth century on Planet Earth, chances are you're well acquainted with anxiety. Overwork, too many decisions to make, too many responsibilities, fear about the future, worries about children, the threat of illness or losing a job, loss of a precious relationship—these are only a few of the potential causes of anxiety in our lives.

Anxiety has a wide range of gradations, from the normal, everyday kind of worries and fears that everyone has, to severe and crippling varieties such as intense panic attacks and phobias. Even the "everyday" kind can be mild or severe. Nervousness before an exam, a job interview, or a first date may be slight or virtually nonexistent for some people, but a source of sleepless nights, sweats, and a palpitating heart for others.

214

Anxiety can be brief and self-limiting—worries about your child's safety that end when he or she finally walks in the door, anxiety about flying that dissipates when you get off the plane—or it can go on for weeks or months. Worries about how to take care of an aging parent, an illness that won't get better, a threatened "downsizing" at work can create anxiety that seems to go on and on.

When anxiety continues for a long time, and/or when it becomes overwhelming and interferes with normal social or occupational functioning, then the situation requires medical attention. But as we will see in this chapter, most common worries and anxieties can easily be treated by oneself, using natural Ayurvedic remedies. And even "serious" anxiety-related disorders can be treated effectively with these same Ayurvedic strategies, though often in conjunction with standard Western modalities such as behavioral therapy or medications.

A Typical Story of Anxiety

Miriam was a notorious worrier. Her children as well as her friends repeatedly tried to point out to her that things never turned out as badly as she imagined they would, but their words had little effect. She was always worried about something or other, and the older she got, the worse it became. She frequently lost sleep over her worries and ended up with a prescription for sleeping pills and another for Valium that she could take when the anxiety became really overwhelming.

Luckily her daughter-in-law recommended an Ayurvedic physician who was able to help Miriam. After evaluating her body type and explaining some Ayurvedic terminology to her, the doctor said, "Worry and anxiety are essentially a disorder of Vata, caused by excess Vata in the system. You have a Vata body type, and both your diet and your daily routine tend to aggravate Vata. This sets you up for a host of Vata-related problems."

It was true; Miriam tended to eat very lightly, including salads of raw vegetables several days a week for lunch, and snacks of dried fruit, both of which increase Vata. Thinking she was doing the right thing in following the usual advice to stay away from fats, she used almost no oil in her diet, though it is important for people with Vata constitutions to have some oil. She also tended to stay up late, watching the 11:00 o'clock news and then staying up at least another hour or more. Both late hours and TV watching tend to aggravate Vata.

In addition, the doctor explained, "Vata tends to increase as we age. At this stage of life, everyone has to start paying attention to balancing Vata. Otherwise, Vata conditions such as dry skin, insomnia, constipation, and yes, increased worry and anxiety, will start to show up more and more."

The doctor prescribed a Vata-balancing regimen for Miriam, including the Vata-pacifying diet and a daily oil massage and suggested diffusing a Vata-soothing aroma in her apartment. The doctor said, "I want you to go to bed earlier and cut out the late-night TV. If you can't sleep, rub your feet for five or ten minutes with a little warm sesame oil."

Making the dietary changes was easier than dropping the long-standing habit of watching TV. But Miriam found that the more she followed the recommendations, the better she felt, so she kept working at it. She felt relieved right away, and within a couple of months much of her anxiety seemed to have vanished; life felt much more comfortable.

This story shows some of the common causes and solutions to anxiety. Let's look more deeply and see what you can do to live a more worry-free life.

What Causes Anxiety?

Anxiety is a mind-body response to a situation that is stressful or perceived as stressful. It's perfectly normal and healthy to feel fear if you see a car heading into your lane; the adrenalin rush and heightened alertness will help you deal with it. Similarly, there are many other everyday situations that can elicit fear and anxiety—concerns about your health, your job, certain family members, living or working in a tense or hostile environment, disturbing news reports or movies, and many more.

Although it's common to feel some anxiety, it's also true that any worry or anxiousness tends to upset our balance. It reduces our enjoyment of the present and cuts down on our ability to deal effectively with what we need to do. And if anxiety persists for a long time or becomes overwhelming, it becomes a serious problem. Some of these more severe forms of anxiety include

- *Panic attacks*: sudden and overwhelming fear, accompanied by symptoms such as shortness of breath, dizziness, rapid heartbeat, nausea, choking sensation, etc.
- *Phobias*: these include so-called "social" phobias, such as fear of social situations like public speaking and "simple" phobias such as fear of heights, open spaces, enclosed spaces, etc.
- *Obsessive-compulsive disorders*: persistent, obsessive thought patterns, often leading to compulsive, repetitive behaviors that one doesn't really want to do but feels compelled to do, such as repeated cleaning or hand washing in order to "avoid" getting some dreaded disease.
- *Post-traumatic stress disorder:* recurrent fearful nightmares or flashbacks that occur *after* some traumatic experience such as a threat to the life of oneself or loved ones, war, or natural disasters such as tornadoes, earthquakes, or floods, acts of violence such as rape, etc.

From an Ayurvedic point of view, we can generalize and say that anxiety is the main Vata response to stress. People with Pitta constitutions generally respond to stress with irritation, anger, and perhaps violence; Kaphas respond with withdrawal and depression. Because anxiety belongs primarily to the domain of aggravated Vata, the recommendations we will discuss in this chapter largely revolve around creating or restoring balance to Vata.

The ancient Ayurvedic texts also mention genetic factors (they speak of "familial" influences), illness, fear of not being able to fulfill one's desires, and overidentification with the past or future as further causes of anxiety.

Ways We Cope with Anxiety

Because our mind-body system tends naturally toward being in balance (or homeostasis), we spontaneously tend to develop our own "self-treatments" for anxiety. Many mental and/or physical diversions, and many good and bad, healthy and unhealthy habits and addictions result from this natural coping mechanism.

Some people develop "good" habits such as sports, reading, or visiting friends, and take up hobbies like knitting, collecting, or working on cars. Others, unfortunately, fall into unhealthy habits often harmful to themselves and/or others, such as habitual or compulsive sex, drug and alcohol abuse, and workaholism, in the effort to avoid the anxiety. A modern common coping mechanism, watching television, can be either positive or negative, depending on how many hours you spend in front of the tube and whether the programs you watch have some educational or uplifting value or are just escapes.

A Dozen Effective Strategies to Reduce or Eliminate Anxiety

Jane was a 28-year-old woman who suffered from occasional panic attacks. These got even worse when she became pregnant. She had been taking medications to help her deal with the attacks, but didn't want to use them while pregnant for fear of hurting her child with the powerful chemicals. Yet at the same time she was terrified of going off the medications because of the almost intolerable attacks of anxiety and fear that could occur seemingly out of nowhere.

At a visit to an Ayurvedic health center, Jane was given more recommendations than she could possibly follow, with the suggestion that she try them and do the ones that felt best and seemed most effective for her. The suggestions follow, pretty much in the order of their importance. Keep in mind that these same recommendations would be helpful—and would be prescribed—for a far less severe case of everyday worries. Try them if anxiety is a problem in your life.

• *Meditate.* Anxiety inevitably brings with it a flood of thoughts and the inability to "shut off the mind." It's very difficult if not impossible to concentrate and focus at school or work, or to settle down at night and fall asleep. The racing mind throws up thousands of thoughts and images, projections of "what might happen," and so on.

One of the best ways to quiet the mind and settle the whole body is to meditate. A number of effective meditation techniques are widely available, and you should learn one and use it regularly! "Mindfulness" meditation is one good choice. Another is "progressive relaxation," which I explained in Chapter 4.

As you've seen throughout the book, I always give my top recommendation to Transcendental Meditation (TM), which has been extensively researched, taught to millions of people, and found to be very effective. A major scientific study comparing TM with other methods of relaxation and meditation found that TM was *twice* as effective in reducing anxiety.

• *Get on a regular routine.* One of the best ways to bring Vata into balance is to develop a more orderly lifestyle. Try to get up and go to bed at about the same time every day, including weekends. Take meals at regular times. Meditate, and do your exercises, at set times. This doesn't mean being fanatical about it. Life doesn't always cooperate with our plans. But you will find that living in this more orderly fashion, creating and following a healthful daily routine (see Chapter 6), will help both your mind and body to be more settled. Problems with anxiety should naturally diminish.

• *Go to bed early.* The key to a healthful daily routine is an early bedtime. Try to be in bed by 10:00, or as close to that as you can make it. Staying up late is one of the best ways to throw Vata out of balance.

• *Follow the Vata-pacifying diet.* The dietary recommendations in Chapter 3 for balancing Vata will work wonders toward reducing anxiety. Avoid cold food and cold or iced drinks. Don't eat many salads, though they're okay in moderation if you use an oily dressing. Avoid dried fruits, apples and pears (both okay cooked), stay away from beans (tofu is okay), and minimize white potatoes and vegetables in the cabbage family such as cabbage, broccoli, and brussels sprouts unless they're well-cooked. Most grains are not good for Vatas: barley, corn, millet, rye, oats should be used sparingly and never in dry form (such as granola).

On the positive side, favor warm foods and drinks, oily food, and food with the three Ayurvedic tastes of sweet, sour, and salty. Rice is good for Vatas, and wheat products are excellent in numerous variations, such as cooked cereals like cream of wheat, pasta, and bread. All dairy products are good for Vatas. Drink milk warm, not cold.

All sweeteners are on your "yes" list, except white refined sugar, which should be off everyone's list. All oils are also good for balancing Vata.

You can eat sweet juicy fruits (grapes, oranges, pineapples, berries, peaches, melons, and more). Among vegetables, most are okay if well cooked, but your best bets are beets, carrots, asparagus, and sweet potatoes. Nuts are a good snack for you (as well as sweet fruit and various sweet desserts). Good spices for Vata include cinnamon, cardamom, ginger, cumin, cloves, salt, and a little black pepper.

• *Daily oil massage.* The Ayurvedic oil massage described in Chapter 4 is a marvelous method for soothing Vata. Follow the directions on pages 58–60. It's easy to learn, enjoyable to do, and produces a wonderful settling effect that lasts through the day. The balanced feeling it creates is a kind of psychological immunity; when you feel centered, things don't bother you easily. This is very helpful for people prone to anxiety.

A related process, which you can't do at home but can have as part of a "panchakarma" purification treatment at an Ayurvedic health center, is known as *shirodhara.* This consists of lying on a specially prepared table (like a massage table) and having warm sesame oil slowly poured in a thin stream onto your forehead.

This may sound strange, but it is one of the most soothing experiences you will ever have. Sharon, a fiftyish woman with severe anxiety and insomnia, had immediate and almost miraculous benifits from a shirodhara treatment. It settled her whole system in just one session, and was helpful in breaking the cycle of long-standing Vata imbalance.

• *Understand your situation.* If you have anxiety symptoms and go to most Western doctors, including mental health practitioners, they may have very little to tell you about why you are feeling that way and what you can do about it. You'll be given a prescription for some tranquilizers, and, depending on your symptoms, you may be urged to do some therapy. If your symptoms are severe, you'll be told that you suffer from a psychiatric illness known as an "anxiety disorder." This will not help you feel good about yourself or your situation!

On the other hand, Ayurveda offers a simple and nonthreatening explanation. Anxiety is primarily caused by Vata imbalance. Certain lifestyle factors aggravate Vata, and others bring it into balance. So if you suffer from anxiety, you need to minimize the causes of imbalance (late hours, erratic schedule, exposure to cold or wind, overwork, too much rushing around, too much sex for your constitutional type, wrong diet, etc.) and maximize the factors that promote balance (regular schedule with early bedtime, Vata-pacifying diet, keeping warm, and all the other factors in this section.)

This understanding of your situation completely avoids the stigma of "having a disease" or being a person with a "mental disorder." It also gives you a sense of direct and realistic control over your situation. You know exactly what to do to help yourself get better. You can do it yourself, starting right now. Even if you have a genetic predisposition toward anxiety, you can still favor the diet and other behaviors that can prevent or reduce the symptoms.

• *Use Vata-balancing herbs.* The following herbs are helpful for balancing Vata and reducing anxiety symptoms: anise, asafoetida, cinnamon, cumin, ginger, gotu kola, licorice, natural sugar, nutmeg, rock salt, sesame seeds, and valerian. The Ayurvedic herbs *ashwagandha, jatamamsi,* and *shankapushpi* are also helpful.

Most of these herbs, such as cinnamon, ginger, and cumin can be used in daily cooking to help pacify Vata. Licorice root and ginger make excellent teas.

Gotu kola is especially helpful for calming the mind and soothing and strengthening the nervous system. It can be taken in capsule form or as a tea.

Valerian, which can be somewhat dulling to the mind, is nevertheless, according to Drs. Vasant Lad and David Frawley in *The Yoga of Herbs,* "one of the best herbs for Vata nervous disorders." It is grounding and soothing and thus is helpful for combating insomnia by gently inducing sleep. You can buy it in capsules or powder form.

• *Follow the Golden Mean.* People with excess Vata in their system frequently tend to overdo it. Balanced Vata increases liveliness and enthusiasm, but aggravated Vata leads easily to excess. People with unbalanced Vata just don't know when to stop, whether at work, at play, cleaning the house, working in the garden, and so on. So remember: Moderation in activity is your golden rule.

This applies to sex as well. You might think that making love would be soothing and settling and thus be good for reducing anxiety, and up to a point you are right. But too much sex for your constitutional type (see Chapter 18) makes Vata imbalance worse and can end up increasing your anxiety.

• *Slow down.* When Vata is out of balance, people not only tend to overdo it in activity, they also tend to rush around at a kind of frenzied pace. Take it a little more easy! Rushing tends to make us less careful and less able to focus, so tasks may actually take *longer* to do than if we worked (drove, cleaned, cooked, etc.) at a more relaxed pace. Rushing can be a product of anxiety, but it can also produce it. So get hold of yourself and settle down. For example, if you are in the habit of walking too fast, make a conscious effort to go at a more relaxed pace.

• *Breathe away your worries.* An effective way to settle your whole system and reduce anxiety and worry is through Ayurvedic breathing. You might try five minutes of balanced, alternate-nostril breathing (see Chapter 4). Or just sit quietly for a few minutes with eyes closed and follow your breathing with your attention. Don't try to change anything; just "watch" the in breath and the out breath. You'll find this very relaxing.

• *Let music soothe away your fears.* A wonderful way to allow anxiety to melt away is to listen to some beautiful music. Pick some music that you find not only enjoyable but also soothing and settling. Sit where you can be really comfortable, or lie down. Close your eyes and just go with the flow. You might find that you get so relaxed you fall asleep. When you wake up, I'll bet you feel much better.

Some suggestions for music include Indian classical music ("Gandharva Veda"), or the slow movements of Western classical pieces. Some New Age music can also have a soothing quality.

• *Fill the air with sweetness.* Our sense of smell affects us strongly. Some fragrances are particularly good for producing a calming and relaxing effect. You can burn incense sticks if you like them, or, for longer-lasting and less smoky effects, diffuse some aroma oil into the air.

There are various kinds of aroma diffusers, available in "New Age" or natural food stores, or by mail (See Appendix C). Some of these work by putting a few drops of oil in warm water. Or, as mentioned in a previous chapter, you can put a few drops of scented oil in a crock pot three quarters full with water and let the scent diffuse through your room or office. In particular, the scents of frankincense, basil, orange, and clove are good for soothing Vata. MAPI products (see Appendix) has a ready-made blend called Vata Oil.

Combat Anxiety by Connecting with Your Deepest Self

According to Maharishi Ayur-Veda, the root cause of anxiety is becoming disconnected from our deepest self, which is said to be a field of bliss or great contentment. When we're in tune with it, centered, we feel at peace. When we're out of touch with it, we start to feel restless and look around outside us for happiness.

When this happens, we lose the ability to live in the present and enjoy it. We worry about the future, or we are gripped by our past and can't let go of it—or we feel it won't let go of us.

In post-traumatic stress disorder, for example, a person is haunted by memories and impressions from painful events in the past. Many Vietnam veterans returned home only to find their lives shadowed for decades by horrible memories of the war. (See Chapter 16.) In phobic disorders, people become afraid that the future will bring some terrible negative outcome. In both these conditions, enjoyment of the present gets sacrificed.

The same is true of less extreme everyday anxieties. We worry about the future. "How will it work out? What will I do? What will he say?" We see a thousand ways for failure, loss, difficulty. Or we play mental and emotional reruns of past experiences. Or we become attached to objects outside ourselves, driving ourselves crazy desiring something we can't have. Or we get what we desire and then become afraid of losing it.

The solution is to reconnect, through quiet meditation, with our inner self, the spiritual aspect of who we are. This is the inner reality of our life, a part of us that is free from all worry and anxiety, an inner sanctuary of peace and contentment. This is the experience of "transcending," going beyond the activity and rigamarole of ordinary daily life to a field of pure, silent consciousness that lies at the deepest level of our own mind.

By regularly alternating this inner silence with activity, we begin to integrate the inner and the outer. We feel more centered, connected to something stable and full inside. This builds a kind of immunity against worry and anxiety, because the more calm, relaxed, and secure we feel in the present, the less we will worry about either the past or the future. The happier we are, the more we can appreciate the moment. We feel more comfortable with our life and with ourself.

So, in a sense, the ultimate cause of anxiety is not being satisfied, not feeling contented. Our mind reaches into the future, re-
works the past, dreams up things to desire, places to go, experiences to have . . . all because we don't feel content in the present.
We become slaves to these desires, to our boredom and our restless, agitated minds.

But wisdom tells us that genuine, lasting satisfaction, security,
and peace of mind can never come from outside. Although we all
have our goals and responsibilities and should do our best to attain
and fulfill them, ultimately we must learn to find solace within. No
matter what we achieve or attain, there will always be something
more to reach for, there will always be the fear of losing what we
have.

In the ancient Vedic tradition from which Ayurveda comes, the
nature of the self is said to be eternal, unchangeable, unbounded. It
is described again and again as a field of bliss and peace. Even a
glimpse of that reality, the ancient sages say, eliminates great fears.

HAPTER 16

HOW TO KEEP YOUR COOL— AYURVEDIC STRATEGIES FOR MASTERING ANGER

Anger can have unfortunate results for everyone involved. If I express anger toward you, it hurts us both. You will feel emotionally bruised by my outburst, but at the same time, the biochemistry that goes along with feeling and expressing anger can do as much harm to me as it does to you—maybe even more. Why is this so?

As we've discussed, research in mind-body medicine is revealing that our body and mind are closely interlinked. For any "event" in one, there is a corresponding activity in the other. When we are angry, not only do we spew out negativity to someone else, but our own body chemistry changes, and these changes can be harmful to our health. Aggressive, hostile behavior patterns have been closely linked by modern medicine with heart disease.

So when you explode or get yelled at by an angry person, it's not just feelings that get wounded; those angry or hurt feelings get

225

translated into a biochemistry of pain that produces stress on your body. In addition, they produce emotional scars that can last a lifetime. So both people suffer negative mental, emotional, and physical consequences.

From the Ayurvedic perspective, anger is not our natural condition; it arises out of physical and mental imbalance. The solution or antidote to anger is to create for ourselves and our loved ones a mind-body system that is healthy, happy, and so balanced that impulses of anger simply don't arise. Creating that ideal state of balance is exactly what Ayurveda sets out to do for every person.

In this chapter, you'll learn some very useful and effective strategies you can use to maintain or restore balance in body and mind, and to release anger in a safe and healthy way. These tips will help prevent anger and all its negative, life-damaging consequences from troubling your life.

Managing Anger with Ayurveda

Ed is a 45-year-old partner in a small insurance office in a midwestern city. Due to a growing conflict with his longtime partner over how to run the company, plus his own tendency to get very wound up and tense at work, Ed has been taking tranquilizers for several years, prescribed by his family doctor. He is usually able to rein in his frustration during the day, but by the time he gets home, despite the medications, he frequently loses his patience and explodes at his family.

Ed's wife had been reading a book on Ayurveda and encouraged him to see a local M.D. with specialized training in Maharishi-Ayur-Veda. Ed was reluctant, but decided to check it out.

When the doctor took Ed's pulse, he told him he had a predominantly Pitta constitution. "That's substantiated by how you look: some baldness early in life, medium build, fair skin. Are you pretty competitive by nature?"

Ed said he was very ambitious.

"Under a lot of stress at work?"

"More than I'd like," said Ed.

"And you're likely to respond by getting irritated easily, maybe having anger outbursts, right?"

Ed laughed. "You can tell that *already?*"

"It goes with the Pitta," the doctor said.

Ed felt immediate relief when he realized he wasn't "going crazy" or "out of control." Rather, he learned he was prone to be a certain way, due to his constitutional makeup. And he was even more relieved when he learned that there were concrete, specific steps he could take to counteract and balance these tendencies.

On the next visit, Ed's wife came along, to learn how she could assist Ed on his journey to becoming a balanced, rather than a "raging" Pitta personality. After all, as her Ayurvedic book said, people with a *balanced* Pitta constitution are supposed to be charming, intelligent, self-confident, passionate, and romantic, as well as excellent leaders. She knew Ed had many of these qualities—but his anger often made her forget.

Ed found out that one major contributing factor to his tendency toward irritability was his diet. He frequently ate fish, and dishes with a lot of cheese (such as pizza). He loved spicy Italian, Mexican, and Indian dishes when he could find them. All of these aggravate Pitta.

Fortunately, his chief cook (his wife) immediately grasped the relationship between diet and behavior. Following the Ayurvedic guidelines, she started to prepare more meals with well-cooked vegetables, rice, and mung beans (small lentils, excellent for Pitta body types). She also made sure to have lots of sweet fruit around the house, such as pears, mangoes, and melons.

She encouraged Ed to take time off to eat a good lunch. Usually he felt he was too busy and had a tendency to skip lunch or put it off till late in the afternoon—a real "no-no" for Pittas.

The doctor also helped Ed realize that he wasn't getting enough exercise. He usually met an old college buddy for a fierce game of racquetball on Saturday morning. But he was essentially sedentary the rest of the week. This all-or-nothing exercise program was setting him up for a heart attack. Just as bad, getting no exercise during the rest of the week was allowing his stress to get too bottled up, without a healthy outlet. Sometimes the cap on the bottle just blew off and Ed erupted in anger.

The doctor told him that exercise, for maximum benefit for him, should be done regularly and should be moderate rather than intensive. High-action sports like racquetball suited his highly competitive temperament and seemed to help him release his aggressions, but there were other types of exercise that would actually be more balancing for him. Swimming would be especially good, as it would have a cooling effect on his system, helping to prevent his hot temper from "overheating."

He also learned some yoga exercises. His wife and his oldest daughter were taking a yoga class. Until his visit to the Ayurvedic doctor, Ed tended to tease them about it, making jokes about "pretzels" and what would happen if they got stuck . . . but when he started to do some of the postures along with them at home a few times a week, to his surprise he found them very calming as well as enlivening.

At the doctor's urging, Ed was also able to fit in a daily oil massage with coconut oil, prior to his morning shower. He expressed amazement that "such a simple thing" could be so helpful in reducing his tendency to become irritable during the day.

These lifestyle changes helped Ed to feel less stressed at work and to be a much more congenial companion at home. Although his tendency toward anger didn't completely disappear overnight, it was, according to his business partner and everyone in his family, greatly reduced.

Ed's story illustrates that the symptoms of anger and irritability, which are extremely common in our society, can be effectively treated through natural approaches.

Understanding the Causes of Anger Can Help Heal It

If we can understand something, we are well on the way to healing it. So it's worth spending a few minutes gaining some deeper knowledge of why we get angry. Then we will go on to a set of strategies to reduce and dissolve anger.

Anger basically has two components, psychological and physiological, that is, mental/emotional causes and physical causes. As we have seen, the two components are closely linked. When a person gets angry, substantial biochemical changes occur in the body. Various chemicals are secreted in the limbic system of the brain, which then communicates to the hypothalamus and the pituitary gland, telling them to release a variety of hormones.

These hormones in turn affect many of the body's organ systems. Blood pressure and pulse increase, acidity in the stomach increases, and many other changes take place. (Interestingly, when a person misses a meal and acidity increases in the stomach, this produces activation of the limbic system—often resulting in anger.)

Anger can occur due to physical causes such as stress; fatigue; illness; lack of exercise; too much exercise; Pitta-increasing foods such as eggs, fish, sour, salty, and spicy foods, and so on. Hot, humid weather conditions—which have been scientifically associated with increased crime—are terrible for people with Pitta body types and can lead to eruptions of anger or violence.

Psychological causes of anger usually involve slights to the ego, in which a person experiences rejection, blame, or a sense of being treated unfairly. Frustration and anger also may result when we fall short of achieving our goals. We may be angry at others for thwarting us, or at ourselves for our perceived shortcomings or for not performing up to the level we expect of ourselves. This is a tendency that perfectionistic Pitta types are prone to have.

From the Ayurvedic perspective, anger has all these causes, but there is a deeper analysis, emphasized by Maharishi-Ayur-Veda, that is useful to know. In this view, anger is the result of not being stationed in Self-knowledge.

So long as our mind is overly attached to attaining happiness from sources outside ourselves, we're bound to become dissatisfied. After all, we can't always get what we want. When we don't, the frustration tends to turn into anger. And even when we do, nothing is permanent. Business gains can turn to losses; someone who loved us yesterday may be gone tomorrow. This, too, can turn to anger.

There is an illuminating verse in the classic Indian scripture *Bhagavad Gita* that shows how overattachment to individuals, outcomes, or situations leads to anger. "Pondering on the objects of the senses," the verse says, "a man develops attachment to them. From attachment springs up desire, and desire gives rise to anger."

Desire leads to anger when it doesn't get fulfilled, or when the desired gain is later lost. A few verses later, the solution is presented: "He whom all desires enter as waters enter the ever-full and unmoved sea attains peace."

In other words, if we are feeling full, happy, and at peace within ourself, then we will not become overly attached to any object of desire. Contented in ourself, we won't feel compelled to reach out to anyone or anything in order to be happy or to achieve a sense of well-being. That doesn't mean we will just sit like a bump on a log, totally unmotivated. Rather, we can act to help others, since we already feel happy inside. We can act *from* a state of well-being, rather than do things in order to reach it.

Everyone's experience shows that when we feel more happy and peaceful within, we naturally see others in a more favorable light. We are less competitive, less demanding, more tolerant and appreciative, more able to empathize. Better understanding and appreciation of what others are going through helps us feel concern for them and makes us less likely to take things personally. The better we feel, the less susceptible we are to slights and "threats" from others. We realize that others are having a hard time, too. They may be blowing off steam from their own built-up stress, not attacking us personally.

Learning how to stay centered in the Self allows us to become increasingly stable and unshakable, like an ocean that barely notices the streams flowing into it. Meditation practiced regularly, along with the other Ayurvedic recommendations in this book, helps us to accomplish this. One of the central concerns of Maharishi Ayurveda is to develop this inner gyroscope, so that the vicissitudes of life don't shake us or throw us over.

Twelve Ayurvedic Strategies to Reduce Anger

Because anger has two components—mind and body—it is practical and intelligent to approach it from both of those sides. This is precisely what Ayurveda does. Some of the following techniques involve the body (exercise, diet, etc.) and some primarily involve the mind (music, meditation). If you put these suggestions to use, you should be able to get a handle on anger.

1. *Listen to soothing music.* In Ayurveda, music has traditionally been used to soothe the mind. Listening to music is helpful for anxiety and insomnia and can also be used to settle angry feelings. You can use any music you find soothing, but for maximum effect, you need to really *listen,* not have the music on in the background. Sit or lie quietly with eyes closed and allow your mind to flow with the sounds. Maharishi Ayur-Veda recommends listening to classical Indian music, especially tunes (raga) that are calming to Pitta. For the best effect listen during the Pitta time of day—10 A.M. to 2 P.M. and around 10 P.M.

2. *Daily oil massage.* As described in Chapter 4, a brief full-body self-massage with a little warm oil can help you immunize yourself against stress. It is calming, settling, and nourishing to mind and body. Remember: Pitta types (the people most prone to anger and irritability) should use coconut oil, which has a cooling effect.

3. *Special nose drops.* Use a sterile eye dropper to place a few drops of warm liquefied ghee in each nostril in the morning. Ghee is one of the most Pitta-pacifying of all substances. Be sure to include some in your diet, too.

4. *Follow the Pitta-balancing diet.* If you are prone to anger outbursts, following the Pitta-pacifying diet should help you, no matter what your body type. One of the major causes of anger is imbalanced Pitta in the system.

If you have a Pitta constitution, following the Pitta diet is essential to keep you healthy and balanced. The diet is described in detail in Chapter 3 but here are a few reminders.

Minimize the sour, salty, and spicy tastes, and instead favor foods that are sweet, bitter, and astringent. Remember, sweet foods include fruit, rice, wheat products such as bread and pasta, and most dairy foods; products made with refined white sugar are not recommended.

Favor cool food and drinks. Salads are good for Pittas, as are most vegetables including asparagus, potatoes, broccoli, cauliflower, green beans, sweet potatoes, and some beans, including kidney beans and soy beans (and soy products such as tofu). Avoid onion, garlic, and hot peppers.

Favor sweet (not sour) fruit; citrus fruit such as grapefruits and lemons may not be for you, but try sweet oranges and see how you feel. Good spices for Pitta include coriander, cinnamon, cardamom, turmeric, cilantro, mint, and small amounts of black pepper.

All sweeteners are all right except honey and molasses, which are heating. Chicken, shrimp, and turkey are acceptable in small amounts, though a vegetarian diet is recommended. Pittas do very well on a vegetarian diet. Avoid alcohol and coffee, which are both very aggravating to Pitta.

5. *Meditate.* Meditation is one of the best ways to defuse stress and prevent it from building up into anger. Here is a story that illustrates that.

Gary was a Vietnam veteran working as a bus mechanic for the city of Denver. Due to his war experiences, Gary was suffering from post-traumatic stress disorder, which manifested itself in extreme anxiety and sudden outbursts of anger. Although he was doing his best to support his wife and son, his violent temper had gotten him fired from several jobs and he was on the verge of losing another when he agreed to participate in a study at the Denver VA hospital. As part of the study, he learned the Transcendental Meditation (TM) technique.*

I moved around a lot when I was a kid and went through six step-mothers. Really—six! It was pretty rough. One of them even shot at me. Then I was shot at in Vietnam for another fifteen months. I was pretty nervous before I went to 'Nam, but when I got back I was strung out, threw fits, yelled all the time. It was hard to hold a job. I got mad real easy. I didn't have much tolerance.

I'm a mechanic and lost jobs because of my temper. I threw things. I used to drink a pint and a half of wine before bed just to help me get to sleep.

One day my supervisor started to talk to me about my being in a bad mood. I pushed him and got canned—actually, I got put on probation. They gave me three months to get my act together, if I went to treatment at the vet center.

They diagnosed me as having "delayed stress syndrome" and told me about a "new program" I could try that was supposed to be good for reducing stress. I didn't know anything about that TM kind of stuff. I was afraid it was a religious cult. I certainly had my doubts about it. But for lots of reasons I tried it. I needed my job, for one thing. And they said there was lots of scientific proof that it worked.

Well, after just a few meditations, maybe a couple of days, I felt a lot better. I was suddenly more in control of myself. I started sleeping better. And after a while, I found I didn't get upset. Things got a lot better at home.

TM was peaceful. Not all the time, mind you. I just felt good after. Now, I may get tired and burned out after a long day, but I never get mad. It happens naturally. I just don't have any animosity.

I think TM gets rid of bad things that have happened. Stressful things. It's just gone.

I have more energy, and I get things done faster. I used to be a fast mechanic, but now I'm even faster. It increases mental aptitude and sharpness all around.

---

*Any veteran can now learn the TM technique free of charge at Veterans Administration (VA) hospitals in the United States, if it is prescribed by a VA doctor.

Because Transcendental Meditation is such an outstanding stress-management tool, it's great for reducing anger and the tendency toward anger.

6. *Follow nature's rhythms.* Some Ayurvedic guidelines for living in tune with nature can help you manage your anger. For example, note that in warmer weather, Pitta tends to become aggravated. This is especially true on days that are both hot and humid, weather many Pittas find virtually intolerable. You have to be even more vigilant about sticking to the Pitta-balancing diet in the summer months. Also, avoid hot showers or overheating from exercise or any other cause. Physical heat and emotional heat are often found together.

As far as your daily routine goes, try to eat a good lunch right around noon, at the height of the daily Pitta cycle. Skipping meals can make Pittas irritable if not downright irascible. And remember to do your coconut oil massage in the morning.

7. *Surround yourself with order and beauty.* As much as you can, spend some time in pleasant, natural surroundings every day. Go for a walk in the woods, around a lake, or in a park. Or at least have some flowers in your office or home. Beauty, order, and natural surroundings are settling to Pittas.

8. *Use herbs for balance.* Most of the herbs I mentioned in the section on diet are good to use in cooking. You can sprinkle fresh cilantro leaves on top of many foods such as curries and other vegetable dishes. Other herbs are effective and often quite delicious as teas. Among these are licorice root (available in teabags in most natural food stores), and a mixture of coriander and fennel seeds. Boil a teaspoon of the seeds in two cups of water until only one cup remains; let it cool before drinking. Or instead of cooking, let a teaspoon of seeds sit in one cup of water overnight, then strain and drink in the morning.

Other teas: Try *Pitta Tea,* a packaged Maharishi Ayur-Veda product that includes several of the herbs I've mentioned. Mint tea (peppermint and/or spearmint) is also cooling and good for Pitta.

An effective Pitta-balancing herb is the Indian herb *shatavari,* or Indian asparagus. Gotu Kola is also helpful and highly recommended if you are very stressed or the anger is combined with a lot of anxiety or irritability.

A final suggestion: Take a tablespoon of aloe vera juice three times a day. Try to get pure juice, sold in natural food stores, not a cheaper diluted brand or one with preservatives.

These herbal remedies are not habit-forming or addictive, and if used properly they have no negative side effects.

9. *Cancel out the caffeine.* Pittas (and Vatas too) should avoid caffeine in all forms, including coffee, tea, and soft drinks.

10. *Use love to combat anger.* Spend some time every day in the company of loving, supportive friends or family members. This is very important to help highly competitive, hard-driving Pitta types relax.

11. *Do your yoga exercises and sun salutations.* A "set" of yoga postures performed each day for about ten or fifteen minutes provides a sense of calm and balance that lasts for hours. It also gives the system an internal massage and stretches the muscles, helping to dissolve stored-up stress.

One posture that is particularly helpful for relieving stress is the shoulder stand. See the descriptions and drawings in Chapter 7, including the cautions about when it might be better not to do these exercises. You can use the Salutation to the Sun (also see Chapter 7) as your primary aerobic exercise, or just for stretching, but try to do it every day.

12. *Shirodhara.* You can't do this one at home, but if there's an Ayurvedic clinic in your vicinity, make an appointment. This technique, which involves having warm herbalized oil poured gently on your forehead in a steady stream, is a traditional remedy for stress, mental agitation, and irritability.

Five Tips for Quickly Cooling Down Anger

Here are five simple tips to quickly defuse anger. Like the previous points, you can use these as preventive measures on a regular basis, but they are also effective as emergency strategies, to immediately cool you down when you begin to get hot under the collar. When you find yourself starting to feel angry or irritated, use these instant strategies. They will quickly start to balance Pitta and reduce anger and aggravation.

1. Put a cool cloth over your eyes for a few minutes.
2. Drink a glass of cold water.
3. Do balanced breathing. The alternate-nostril breathing exercise called balanced breathing (explained in Chapter 4) is helpful to settle all body types and can be used effectively as an antidote for anger.
4. Eat a small dish of ice cream, or take a spoonful of ghee.
5. Instead of blowing off steam at someone, sit down by yourself, close your eyes, and just stay for a few minutes. During that time, let yourself feel any sensations going on in your body, such as heat or pressure. Just be with it; observe and feel it with neutrality. You'll feel a lot more settled and calm in just a few minutes.

Anger is one of the most devastating of the human emotions. It tears apart the person who feels it, often leaving in its wake guilt and pain for saying and doing things when "out of control" that would never have been said or done under normal circumstances. It also inflicts great pain on those who bear the brunt of the outbursts of rage. How much sweeter and more harmonious human life would be without it!

Ayurveda teaches that anger arises primarily from imbalance and provides many effective, time-tested strategies, including the ones just described, to maintain balance and head off anger before it arises. I hope you will use these simple remedies. They have the power to change your life.

CHAPTER 17

AYURVEDIC SECRETS FOR FULFILLING RELATIONSHIPS

Knowledge of the Ayurvedic body types is invaluable for creating successful, loving relationships. It offers us greater self-understanding—why we act and react the way we do—and at the same time vastly increases our understanding of why the people we are connected to act and react the way *they* do.

The better we understand the constitutional types, the more we realize that people truly are different from one another. And because of these inherent physical and psychological differences, our husbands and wives, our parents and children, our friends and co-workers are not going to be like us.

This one fact—that people are different—is one of the most difficult things to learn in relationships.

Ordinarily, instead of respecting one another's differences, we tend to project our own ideas, values, and ways onto others, and we expect them to be like us. If they're not, we tend to reject them or try to change them. Real constitutional differences are bound to create conflicts, from little things like what temperature to keep the house (Pittas like it cool, Vatas and Kaphas warm) to larger issues such as spending patterns (Vatas are unpredictable, Pittas like luxury, and Kaphas conserve).

When these inevitable conflicts arise, people usually feel that in order for the relationship to improve, *the other person* has to change. He or she has to be more like me. This is a crucial mistake. It is unfair to the other person, and it doesn't work. It only creates resentment and tension.

The best way to resolve such conflicts is through mutual understanding. Learning about our own Ayurvedic mind-body constitutional type and the constitution of those we are close to can help us step out of the trap of trying to make others be like us. If we are ever going to get along harmoniously, to really love and appreciate them for who they are and to know how to help them unfold their unique capabilities, knowledge of their personality types is extremely useful.

The knowledge of body types has helped many couples understand and respect each other's differences and has helped create or restore harmony and love in their lives. It is also helpful to parents. It provides not just the abstract concept, "People are different," but deep knowledge of how they're different.

"Oh, he has a Pitta constitution," a prudent wife might say to herself when she sees her husband getting hot under the collar. "He tends to flare up, and I have just the right thing to help." For a Pitta person, something as simple as a glass of cool water or a small dish of ice cream can short-circuit a potential emotional explosion.

Or a mother might know, "My daughter is Vata. When she comes home from school in a state of agitation, talking so fast I can hardly keep up and unable to settle down to her homework, I can give her a cup of Vata-pacifying tea or some warm soup and toast, which will help soothe the Vata."

Should My Partner Have the Same Body Type?

Traditionally, Ayurveda recommends that for sexual compatibility people of the same constitutional type make the best partners because their sexual appetites and capacities will be matched. We will discuss this at length in the next chapter. But there are other key factors in relationships besides sex, and here the principle of balance comes into play.

Naturally, it will be easier to understand someone whose makeup is similar to your own. But it may not be any easier to get along. Two spacey, talkative, disorganized Vatas may drive each other crazy; two competitive, hot-tempered, hypercritical Pittas could make life miserable for each other. A couple of Kaphas could sink into a life of minimal activity, ending up overweight, under-stimulated, and quite unhappy. There is a lot to be said for living with someone who is your opposite, whose constitutional type will balance, rather than mirror, your own.

Robert Svoboda, a modern Ayurvedic practitioner, teacher, and author has suggested that for comfort and harmony, living with someone like you is best, but for growth, stimulation, and challenge opposites may be better. This may work as a general guideline, but don't forget that every situation is unique.

Differences in personality type can be problematical, but they are also sources of mutual enrichment. Opposites not only attract, they also complement and complete each other. Indeed, it is common for opposites to marry, and in most cases it seems to work well. Just as balance is important for health within each individual, it can also be valuable in a marriage.

For example, a couple in which one person is primarily Vata and the other is Kapha form a good combination. Even better would be a Vata-Pitta and a Kapha-Pitta, who will tend to balance each other and form a stable relationship. The mutual Pitta will create fire, passion, and good communication between them; the Kapha qualities will provide stability for the Vata, and the Vata qualities will stimulate and challenge the Kapha.

A hard-driving Pitta-Vata man named Jim, who had what Western medicine would classify as a Type A personality, is married to Sue, a sweet, easygoing Kapha woman. Sue enjoys Jim's energy and the success he has in his work; Jim feels nourished by Sue's softness, which he badly needs when he comes home from the office. He can act in the world in ways she would never feel comfortable acting, while she offers him stability, patience, and a supportive presence at home. The result is that both achieve a greater balance.

This is very natural. Wholeness within oneself is surely a worthwhile ideal to strive for. But in practical life, if there's an imbalance that one person feels, or a lack of certain qualities or abilities, by putting two together you create a wholeness that is greater than the sum of the parts. Life becomes better for both.

How the Types Interact in Relationships

Now let's take a look at how the personality types interact in intimate relationships. For simplicity, we will deal with only the three main types, Vata, Pitta, and Kapha. But remember: Almost all of us are combinations of these three qualities, so you'll need to adapt these basic definitions in order to understand yourself and how you interact with those close to you.

Suggestion: Before you read further, review the characteristics of the different body types in Chapter 2.

Vatas in Relationships

Vatas are vivacious, communicative, and demonstrative and can bring much delight to relationships. They have a strong need for touch and physical contact, though (as we shall soon see) their sexual stamina is not high, so they are often more comfortable with less sexual activity than the other constitutional types. Balancing Vata dosha helps them become more consistent, less flighty, and less prone to self-doubt. They are thinner-skinned than others, and thus are prone to easily having their feelings hurt.

Vatas with Vatas

This combination can be wonderfully artistic and freewheeling. The only danger is that the household can become chaos. Balancing Vata—by following the Vata-pacifying diet, doing daily oil massage, and striving for a more regular daily routine—helps the partners avoid erratic schedules, missed appointments, sloppiness, and so on.

Vatas with Pittas

Vatas can gain discipline from Pittas and can learn to be neater. But they must realize that Pittas don't always like physical contact as much as they do, and they should not take this as a rejection. Also, Pittas can be direct in their speech and don't necessarily mean to be unkind when they speak in a way that, to the more highly sensitive Vata, may seem harsh.

Vatas like variety in all areas, including friendships, of which they will have many. Pittas, however, get jealous easily, and the Vata spouse's wide-ranging and easy friendliness can sometimes upset them. Mutual understanding here can avoid a lot of bad feelings.

Vatas with Kaphas

The Kapha's slow, steady pace and solid, easy approach to things is a great anchor for the changeable, often erratic Vata. Vata types may tend to become impatient with Kapha slowness, but they can profit from it to slow down their own sometimes frantic pace a bit.

The Vata tendency to a wide variety of friends and acquaintances may baffle the Kapha, who prefers one or two deep, long-lasting friendships.

If you have a Vata partner, it will help you to understand and accept him or her if you remember that Vatas by nature tend to worry, have a hard time keeping to a schedule or routine, crave change and variety, change their minds easily and often, and have their feelings easily hurt.

Pittas in Relationships

Pittas tend to be highly passionate and are ardent romantics when they fall in love, a quality that has rarely hurt any relationship. They are also decisive, so you know where they stand. Their clear thinking, self-discipline, and decisiveness can make them excellent partners in any business situation or in a crisis.

A key Pitta problem is a tendency toward anger. Pitta fuses can be short. If you are a Pitta, to avoid inflicting your anger on those closest to you, take care to balance Pitta dosha: Avoid spicy foods, staying too long in the sauna, too much exposure to the sun, and anything that exacerbates your tendency to "overheat."

Pittas also have a need for beauty and orderliness in their environment that is a double-edged sword—wonderful when it is moderated and produces neat, lovely surroundings, overbearing when it becomes obsessive.

Pittas with Vatas

Pittas, who like things organized and on schedule, can benefit from the loosening up that a relationship with a free-flowing Vata requires. They will have to learn to accept a little disorder in the environment, as well as in daily routines. They will need to be extra watchful of their tempers, as Vatas are easily upset.

As mentioned earlier, Vatas like to have friendships with many people. If a Pitta understands this tendency, it will counterbalance the Pitta propensity toward jealousy.

Pittas with Pittas

Pitta partners will have a mutual understanding of each other, and their ambition and focused energy make a great team for accomplishment. But they will have to be careful to avoid two tendencies that are potentially disruptive to the relationship.

The first is battling each other, which can happen when Pitta dosha gets unbalanced and tempers flare. They will also have a tendency to compete with each other, as Pittas are highly prone to competitiveness. Sticking with a Pitta-balancing routine and practicing a stress-management technique such as TM can help maintain peace in this household.

Pittas with Kaphas

The Kapha's cool, steadying influence is soothing to fiery Pittas. Also, Kaphas are forgiving and easygoing, so they don't take Pitta anger or competitive drive as personally as others. Still, Pittas will have to be on the alert not to lose their tempers when their Kapha partner seems too slow and "laid back"—a danger, since the ambitious Pitta tends to feel intense time pressure. Pitta must learn that Kapha's slow and steady approach often wins the race.

If you have a Pitta partner, it will help you to understand and accept him or her if you remember that Pittas have an inherent tendency to find fault outside themselves and thus to blame those around them for anything that goes wrong. They are usually smart, insightful, and competent and find it difficult to believe that they can also make mistakes. Remember that Pittas, more than the other personality types, crave beauty and neatness in their surroundings. They also like to be on time.

Kaphas in Relationships

Kaphas are affectionate, steady, calm, easygoing, and forgiving—all of which are wonderful qualities to find in a partner. A husband telling his Kapha wife that he's going to spend Saturday at the golf course can expect to hear, "Have a good game, honey"—not necessarily what a Vata or Pitta wife would say.

Three things that Kaphas need to watch out for in relationships, all the results of imbalanced Kapha, are possessiveness, lethargy, and being overly self-contained.

Kaphas with Vatas

This can be an excellent combination, as Vata brightens up the Kapha's life, adding excitement, while the Kapha brings steadiness to the Vata. The main thing to watch out for is conflict between the slow, steady Kapha style and the quick, changeable Vata style.

Vatas like meeting new people and trying new things, while Kaphas tend toward a few steady friendships and a simple, home-centered life. If they are out of balance, a Vata can view a Kapha as a stick-in-the-mud, while a Kapha will see the Vata as running around like a headless chicken. Both gain by accommodating—the Kapha gets around a little more, and the Vata stays a little more grounded.

Kaphas with Pittas

On the plus side, Pittas can add drive, ardor, and ambition to the Kapha's quiet life, while Kaphas offer stability and gentleness to their ambitious Pitta partner. However, this combination is especially at risk for what is known as co-dependency. The mild-mannered and tolerant Kapha often puts up with hypercritical, aggressive, or even abusive behavior in the Pitta, especially when there is an imbalance that accentuates these Pitta qualities.

With repeated instances of this kind of abusive behavior, the Kapha person becomes silently resentful and withdrawn. This withdrawal further annoys and infuriates the Pitta partner, which elicits a deeper withdrawal and increased resentment.

This vicious cycle can be reversed if the couple gains proper understanding of their situation and takes measures—through diet, exercise, and so forth—to get back in balance. In cases of true co-dependency, seeking professional counseling may well be necessary to fully resolve the situation.

Kaphas with Kaphas

This can be a steady, affectionate pairing, whose path to happiness will be smoothed by a mutual patience and acceptance that is entirely natural and unforced. If they're not careful, however, they may reinforce each other's tendencies to get into a rut or become lethargic "couch potatoes." They need to remind each other to exercise, to eat lightly, and to get out of the house and try new things. Responding to invitations from their more adventurous Vata or Pitta friends will help.

If you have a Kapha partner, it will help you to understand and accept him or her if you remember that Kaphas tend to be slow and steady, but their calm persistence will help them to cross the finish line. Be patient with their initial slowness in learning and action. Once they learn, they don't easily forget; once started on a course of action, they don't give up, but tend to complete what they start. They are very loyal and dependable but sometimes can be possessive. Overall, a Kapha partner is consistent, congenial, and tolerant.

How a Difficult Marriage Was Healed Through Understanding Ayurvedic Body Types: A Case History

Now that you have become an expert in the Ayurvedic body types and their corresponding personality traits, it will be easy for you to follow this case history. Use it as a model to help you understand conflicts in your own relationships or to help your friends when they come to you with their problems.

The story of Anne and John, a couple in their late thirties, is told by Dr. Brooks, co-author of this book and a psychiatrist trained in Maharishi Ayur-Veda. It begins when they first visited his office.

"I don't see what can save our marriage," Anne said as soon as she sat down. Her face was thin and pale, and her speech was very rapid. Her husband John, a large, heavyset man, glanced at her but said nothing.

Anne complained that John was unaffectionate. "He doesn't love me," she said. "He just sits there all evening, either in front of the TV, reading, or listening to music. He hardly notices me, and if I try to get his attention, he really doesn't respond. He never tells me he loves me and hardly ever touches me. It's clear that he just doesn't love me anymore."

After getting some background, it became clear to me that here was a classic marriage of opposites. Anne was creative, bright, vivacious, but she was high-strung and easily became upset or anxious. John was very self-contained. Hard-working, quiet, and undramatic, he simply wasn't the demonstrative kind.

Anne spoke freely and at length about their problems, but John said almost nothing. Finally, with much support and encouragement, he began to speak about his perspective on their situation. He said Anne was driving him crazy. "She's so aggravating," he grumped. "You can't have a moment's peace in the house. She's always bustling around doing something or other, or else she talks, talks, talks—you never get a moment's rest."

The tensions had been escalating for several years. By the time the couple went into marriage counseling, their relationship was hanging by a thread. The key to stitching it together more firmly soon emerged, however.

It was apparent that John—heavy, slow, phlegmatic—was predominantly a Kapha personality and that Anne—quick, sensitive, lively—was a Vata. By diagnosis of the pulse and some questioning, it was clear that John also had quite a bit of Pitta in his makeup.

The couple's conflicts were largely a product of failing to understand and accept each other's different natural tendencies. Vata is related to the skin and the sense of touch. Vata types are naturally airy and can be somewhat ungrounded, especially when out of balance. For these reasons, touching is important for them.

Kaphas can be very self-sufficient, and Pittas (John's secondary quality) may actively dislike physical contact. That made John more comfortable with limited touching, and he felt Anne was too demanding in that department; Anne, who craved more physical affection, interpreted John's attitude as rejection.

Both were only being true to their natures, but they didn't realize this. Each felt personally attacked, and each failed to understand the other's needs and tendencies.

Anne's Vata personality was naturally communicative. John was naturally self-contained. Anne needed to talk and interact; John preferred to read or to sit quietly in front of the tube.

Anne was also, as most Vata individuals tend to be, very gregarious and social. Like most Vatas, she hated routine and craved variety in life. She had many friends and moved easily from one friend or social circle to the next. All this was completely normal for someone with a Vata body type.

But it was a problem for John. Kaphas can be very possessive, and John was no exception. Like most Kaphas, he had only a few friendships, but they were very deep. He was much more cautious than Anne in forming relationships, more slow to get to know somebody, but when he made a friend, he was loyal for life.

Kaphas do not readily understand Vatas, who are so different from them, and John did not understand or approve of Anne's social style. He felt a bit threatened by her comfort with many people and many diverse activities, and the Pitta in his personality flared up and made him a little angry. "She flits around too much," he complained.

Anne, of course, reacted by calling John a stick-in-the-mud who always wanted to see the same one or two people, who was a homebody and never wanted to go out.

She felt upset with her husband for being possessive for what seemed to her like no valid reason, and she began to feel closed in and claustrophobic in the relationship. Her Vata nature, to move around and be active, was being suppressed and inhibited.

Anne's worries about the unhappy situation made it difficult for her to relax. She slept badly, and her insomnia threw her Vata further out of balance, increasing her nervousness.

John dealt with his annoyance by eating and watching TV. His overeating and lack of exercise exaggerated his Kapha tendencies, and he became increasingly passive and withdrawn.

The marriage counseling focused on helping each gain a better understanding of the other's basic nature. When they understood what was going on, they were able to break the vicious cycle.

Anne realized, "Ninety percent of this has nothing to do with me. It's John's nature. He was born this way. He'll never be like me. But there's nothing wrong with what he is. It's just different." It was a huge relief to her. She began to recognize that her sense of being rejected was a misinterpretation, a projection of her fears. John was simply undemonstrative by nature; his lack of responsiveness wasn't personally directed toward her.

For John, understanding Anne's inherent liveliness and sociability was a breakthrough too. These insights created an objectivity that let them draw back from the anger and resentment.

The next task was to help them remember why they had been attracted to each other in the first place. Now that they had gotten their resentments out in the open, it was time for healing. I asked them to sit together and to think of all the ways they appreciated each other, then turn to each other and say what those ways were.

Many of the answers they came up with expressed the best qualities of each other's personality type. Anne said, "John's strength and stability attracted me because it provided just the kind of dependable foundation I needed." John said, "What most attracted me about Anne was her vitality, her sparkle." She kept him from getting passive and withdrawn, he said; "she brought adventure and excitement into my life."

These "positive" qualities had innocently attracted them to each other. Later in the relationship, the "negative" qualities—the opposite side of the coin—rose to the surface. Anne's Vata tendencies had once charmed John, but when they got out of control, they drove him batty. John's stability had made Anne feel secure, but then she saw him turning into a couch potato.

They had tears in their eyes as they told each other these things. For the first time in many months, they realized how deeply they loved each other and how much their partner actually did love them.

But there was more to be done. The key to regaining the magic and joy of their early relationship was not only to appreciate their differing natures but also to restore balance within their own bodies. Anything that aggravated Anne's Vata—for example, staying up late—would eventually aggravate her husband as she went spinning and chattering around the house. And when John ate too much pizza or got too little exercise, his Kapha would build up and make him unbearably passive and uncommunicative.

I recommended that John and Anne help each other with the ongoing process of creating balance in their bodies. John's "job" included gently reminding Anne to go to bed on time and to give herself a daily oil massage; he even made it a point to give her a massage himself on a regular basis, which she deeply enjoyed. Anne agreed to help him watch his diet and to remind him to get enough exercise. She signed them both up for tennis lessons. Doing these things made their individual lives better, they explained, and at the same time they also made their relationship more loving.

When Anne and John left the therapy after just a few sessions, they went home armed with a deeper mutual understanding, acceptance, and appreciation and a list of things to do to bring balance to their bodies and minds and harmony to their marriage.

Five Ways You Can Balance Your Body to Build Harmony in Your Relationships

As the story of Anne and John shows, an intellectual understanding about Ayurvedic personality types is helpful, but it's only part of the story of successful relationships. An equally crucial role is played by maintaining health and balance in our bodies.

No matter how much we understand and no matter how much we work on factors such as communication skills, expressing feelings openly, and so forth, if our physical system is out of balance or full of stress that clouds our thinking and upsets our feelings, then all this intellectual knowledge will have only limited value. So it's absolutely critical to keep the body healthy and in balance.

For example, Tom, a 46-year-old man with a Pitta body type, vows to himself on the way home from work, "I'm going to be nice today. Regardless of what the kids do, I'm not going to yell." He is completely sincere. But when he gets home, tired after a difficult day at work and stressed out from an aggravating traffic jam, he finds that his teenaged son didn't take out the trash—again—and the garbage collectors have come and gone for the week. Despite his best intentions, he yells at his son. He's too out of balance to be able to fulfill his vow.

The remedy is quite simple. A few minutes of meditation before he left work or on the bus on the way home would have dissolved much of that stress and fatigue. A cool drink or washing his face in cool water or a regular habit of taking Pitta-reducing herbs would have helped him remain settled, calm, and better able to deal with the situation without flying off the handle.

Here are some other ways you can help maintain balance in your physiology. These will help keep you more centered in yourself, more emotionally stable and happy, and able to be more understanding and giving in all your relationships:

1. Massage: A daily abhyanga (self-massage) increases psychological as well as physical resistance—immunity—so that if you are experiencing a stressful situation, you're less likely to get upset. According to Ayurvedic theory, this is because the massage balances Vata dosha. In Western terms this means that it strengthens the nervous system, which is governed by Vata.

2. Exercise: Another element in strengthening and healing the body is the proper kind of exercise for your constitution. Exercise can reduce stress and promote a feeling of health and confidence. When you feel better you're naturally able to be more loving and patient. It's not surprising that many people find that when they start exercising their relationships improve. "I started jogging and I'm getting along better with my wife."

But you have to do the appropriate type and amount of exercise. Too much can aggravate Vata and make a person with a lot of Vata in his or her constitution feel exhausted and cranky rather than energized. Exercise that's too heating can make Pitta tempers flare. On the other hand, not getting enough exercise aggravates Kapha; if you are a Kapha type, this may result in sluggishness and depression. See Chapter 7 for help in determining the amount and type of exercise that is best for you.

3. Diet: Proper diet is one of the foundations of physical and emotional stability. Food affects our mood, our energy level, and our state of emotional equilibrium.

The first step is to learn your constitutional type. After that, you can easily apply the knowledge of Ayurvedic nutrition in your daily life. This is practical and important because the aggravation of Vata, Pitta, or Kapha due to improper diet can be a major factor in disturbing the harmony we are all seeking in our relationships.

Margaret would sometimes find herself feeling irritable for no apparent reason, snapping at family members and then feeling guilty about it, since there seemed to be no reason for her mood. The feeling would come over her for one or two hours and then would subside just as rapidly as it had come.

By carefully observing her daily habits, including her diet, it became apparent that this occurred approximately half an hour after she ate some fish. Because she knew from her study of Ayurveda that she had a Pitta body type, and fish increases Pitta, she theorized that fish might be causing the problem. Although she was an avid seafood lover, she experimented, cutting back her fish consumption rather sharply. To her family's relief, when she ate less fish, she became a more pleasant companion after meals.

In the same way, foods that aggravate Vata (such as salads, cold foods, dry foods) can make a person of Vata body type more anxious and irritable, and foods that aggravate Kapha (dairy foods, meats, sweets, wheat products) tend to produce dullness and depressed moods in Kaphas. As remarkable as it may sound, simply regulating your diet can help to avoid these imbalances, which in turn can have a major impact on improving your relationships. Refer to the charts on pages 43–49 to choose the foods that promote balance for you.

4. Herbal food supplements: Various herbs and herbal compounds can result in greatly increased emotional stability, along with a strengthening of the body and nervous system. Simply using the herbs and spices listed in the food charts on pages 43–49 when you prepare your meals can help you balance your system. Here are a few examples of individual herbs that may be useful to you, according to your body type:

> **Vata**—anise, asafoetida, cinnamon, cumin, ginger, gotu kola, licorice, natural (unrefined) sugar, nutmeg, rock salt, sesame seeds, and valerian.
>
> **Pitta**—aloe, burdock, chrysanthemum, coconut, coriander, cumin, fennel, golden seal, mint, pomegranate, sandalwood, shatavari (Indian asparagus), natural sugar, and turmeric.
>
> **Kapha**—alfalfa, basil, black pepper, cardamom, cinnamon, cloves, cumin, eucalyptus, fenugreek, garlic, ginger, Indian long pepper (pippali), peppermint, sarsaparilla, spearmint, turmeric, and wintergreen.

The herbal preparations known as rasayanas (rejuvenating tonics) enhance the feeling of well-being and vitality and can thus contribute significantly to the quality of relationships. One such compound, known as chyavanprash, composed of several Ayurvedic herbs, is available from different manufacturers in many natural food stores or from the sources listed in Appendix C. A similar herbal preparation, Maharishi Amrit Kalash, has been researched in the West and appears to be highly beneficial for both mental and physical health.

5. Daily routine: Almost everyone has experienced that we tend to be more irritable and less patient with others when we haven't gotten enough sleep or when we've gone for too long without having something to eat. The suggested Ayurvedic daily routine (see pages 82–85) is the product of centuries of observation of what living patterns keep us most healthy. Simply following a few of the guidelines can keep us in balance and functioning at our best.

In particular, going to bed on time (during the Kapha phase of the daily cycle, before 10:00 P.M.); eating your largest meal for lunch, around 12 noon; performing a daily self-massage with a little oil; and regular practice of an effective meditation technique such as T.M. can provide the clarity, energy, and joyfulness to make the most of our lives and our relationships.

Take Care of Yourself—You're the Center of All Your Relationships

It may be obvious to state this, but the first step in improving any relationship is to improve our ability to give. Maharishi Mahesh Yogi, the founder of the Transcendental Meditation movement and a major figure in the revival of Ayurveda in the twentieth century, has frequently pointed out that if two people meet with the goal of receiving from each other, then no one gives; if no one gives, no one can receive. The fundamental principle in the art of successful, fulfilling relationships, he says, is mutual giving.

However, giving is based on who we are. We can only relate to others, give to others, understand and care for others based on what we are. "Only a lit bulb can give light," Maharishi has said. Because the Self is the center of all relationships, the more fully we mine our own inner reserves of creativity and strength, the better we can see, understand, love, and help others.

So it's not selfish to take time to develop our own abilities, to become all that we can be. In fact it's vital to do so, so that we'll have more to offer. And it's vital that we take good care of ourselves, not neglecting our health. We need to eat well and to get enough rest. This applies to everyone, including those who tend to ignore their own needs, either in the drive for success or in their care or service to others.

Secrets of Dealing with Negative Feelings

Ayurveda, much like modern psychiatry, emphasizes the importance of not bottling up our feelings, as this can lead to stress not only in the mind, but also in the body. The growing understanding of mind-body medicine and psychosomatic illness is based on the recognition that the storing-up of bad feelings causes both mental and physical illness.

You may find it interesting that Sigmund Freud, the founder of modern psychiatry, believed that specific kinds of repressed feelings would give rise to specific mental and/or physical illnesses. This is now being borne out by research, nearly 100 years later. So it's important to find ways to rid ourselves of negativity.

According to Ayurveda, feeling happy and balanced is *normal*. If you have bad feelings, if you are angry, depressed, irritable, anxious, that means that something is out of whack in your system. That doesn't mean you're a bad person—everybody gets out of balance sometimes. Probably you are overtired, or your doshas are out of balance because of stress or something you ate. The trick is to get your equilibrium back. When you are in balance you will feel essentially even, contented, energetic, and happy.

Therefore, it is useful to check in with yourself once in awhile and notice how you're feeling. This is a concept we've talked about before, in conjunction with eating foods that are good for you, and in not eating too much. When you keep an eye on your feelings, then, if something starts to irritate you, frighten you, and so on, you can catch it before the bad feelings build up. Then you can take some action—talk about it, drink an herb tea to calm you, and so on—to correct the situation.

The Ayurvedic sages also strongly emphasize the importance of not expressing negative feelings in a way that harms others. From this standpoint there has been far too much emphasis in the West in recent years on self-expression for its own sake, getting it off your chest and letting someone else have it. This is neither creative nor useful. It simply transfers the pain and reduces trust.

The classical Ayurvedic texts recommend to speak the truth, but to do it "sweetly." Being respectful and tactful in one's speech and behavior is always a good policy.

Four Ways to Free Yourself of Negative Feelings

To resolve this paradox—don't bottle up feelings, but don't dump on the people you love—here are some suggestions. They are not derived specifically from traditional Ayurvedic texts, but are in the spirit of both modern psychology and Ayurveda:

1. Talk about it. If you have pent-up feelings of frustration or anger that frequently come bursting out, it can be helpful to talk with a trusted friend or family member or with a trained counselor. In this way you can often avoid taking out your negativity on those closest to you. Talking allows for the constructive release of these emotions.

2. Try exercise. For chronic (recurrent) as well as acute (immediate) situations, you may be able to release strong negative feelings *by yourself*. One way that many people find helpful is through exercise, such as jogging, working out with weights or an exercise machine, or by doing yoga (see Chapter 7 for exercise recommendations by body type).

3. Let the feelings pour out. You can also go into a room by yourself and allow the feelings to come out. You can do this simply by closing your eyes and just experiencing the feelings for a few minutes; this is often sufficient to reduce or release them. Sometimes pounding a pillow, crying, even screaming (into a pillow if you don't want neighbors or others in the house to hear you) may be helpful in releasing the pent-up emotion. Don't feel embarrassed or ashamed to let yourself do this.

A particularly effective way to dissolve negative feelings is, with eyes closed, to direct your attention to the sensations present in your body. You'll be surprised how simple it is, with this method, to transform your mind from a state of negativity to a state of calmness and inner peace.

After you've released your negative emotions in the privacy of your room and you feel better, you'll be glad you didn't let out your feelings in a hurtful way to someone you love. And you'll be able to talk about what was bothering you, or act on it, with more calm and clarity.

4. Use a stress-reduction technique. One of the best tools for keeping negative feelings from making us act in ways we'd rather not behave is to practice meditation or some other sort of relaxation technique that you find helpful. This acts like a safety valve that releases a little of the stress every day, keeping the pressure from building up inside. There have been a number of published studies indicating that T.M. helps relationships by reducing anger, irritability, fear, and other negative emotions. At the same time it enhances positive feelings like confidence, happiness, and world peace.

You don't have to wait for marriage counseling to make your relationship work. You can avert most problems or resolve them if they arise through the knowledge and techniques in this chapter and throughout the book. Understand the requirements of your own and your partner's constitutional type so that you can intelligently organize your life—your schedule, what you eat, how much and what kind of exercise to get, and so on—to maintain emotional balance. Enlivening the spiritual dimension is especially important.

SEX AND YOUR CONSTITUTIONAL TYPE: AYURVEDIC SECRETS FOR INTIMACY AND FULFILLMENT

Sex is one of the most pleasurable and powerful aspects of life, as it represents the force of life and life's continuity. Sex is as natural a part of living as eating and drinking, and yet, in the modern Western world, it has become a problem for millions of people, widely misunderstood and misused.

In ancient India, which gave birth to the knowledge of Ayurveda, life was much more natural, tied to the earth and the seasons, and sex was more properly understood. Indian culture has long recognized sex as a tremendously vital force and symbolizes this in its traditional art and worship of the Divine Mother (Shakti) as an equal partner of the male aspect of God (Shiva), the two often pictured in sexual embrace, creating the world.

From the Ayurvedic point of view, our culture places far too much emphasis on sex. And our understanding of human sexuality is incomplete and in some important ways incorrect, which has serious repercussions on our mental and emotional health and on our relationships.

In this chapter we'll look at some Ayurvedic principles that can give us a healthier, richer sex life.

254

How Strong is Your Sex Drive?
Sex and Your Ayurvedic Body Type

We Westerners seem to have a universal understanding about sex that boils down to one simple rule: The more the better. But the fact is that individuals have differing degrees of interest in sexual activity and very different degrees of "tolerance" for it.

In a famous scene in Woody Allen's classic film *Annie Hall* the screen splits; on one side we see Woody with his therapist and on the other Diane Keaton with hers. At the same moment, each therapist asks, "How often do you make love?"

> Woody: "Hardly ever. Maybe three times a week."

> Diane: "Constantly. I'd say, three times a week."

As funny as this is in the movie, it points to a reality that is often problematic for couples. Some people desire a great deal of sexual activity, while others—both men and women—are content with much less.

According to Ayurveda, the amount of lovemaking that is comfortable for each person is to a large extent dependent upon constitutional type. Guidelines are provided suggesting what is appropriate for each person.

- **Kaphas** have the strongest sexual "endurance." Just as Kapha types need and enjoy more vigorous physical exercise than Vatas or Pittas, their sexual drive is also greater. Though Kaphas are usually not as "driven" toward sex—it takes them longer to get interested—a Kapha person will typically have a great deal of fortitude and sustaining power in sexual activity and will also tend to feel strong and well after making love.

- **Vatas** generally require the least amount of sex. People with a predominantly Vata body type are generally content and comfortable with the least among the three constitutions. Too frequent lovemaking for their constitution can have an energy-depleting, Vata-aggravating effect. This will lead to typical Vata disorders such as anxiety, insomnia, or weakness of the nervous system. Excess sex—for his or her constitution—will make the Vata person very tired.

- **Pittas** have an intermediate sexual drive. Even though they are often fiery, romantic, and passionate, Pittas don't tolerate as much sexual activity as Kaphas.

Regarding sexual compatibility, the best matches are generally between people of the same constitutional type. Their sexual appetites and capacities are similar; they will understand each other and have similar needs and desires. People with very different sexual needs may find their relationships severely strained.

A Vata person with a Kapha partner, for example, may find himself or herself exhausted, or resentful of the partner's continuing sexual demands. For the Vata, infrequent lovemaking can be quite normal and will be comfortable both psychologically and physically. On the other hand, the Kapha partner in this match might be perpetually unfulfilled sexually due to the Vata's lukewarm interest.

Another problem for this couple is likely to come from the fact that Kaphas are slower to be aroused, but once they get warmed up, they typically sustain their desire and like to continue making love for a long time. Vatas, on the other hand, are quickly excited and quickly finished. If the Vata partner is a man, he will have a tendency toward what our culture considers to be "premature ejaculation," simply because he's Vata. He will have considerable difficulty sustaining intercourse for a long period of time, and this will make him feel inadequate, especially when a Kapha friend brags about how long he can go on.

Although a Vata man will always have this tendency, he can reduce it somewhat by following a Vata-balancing diet, living a more regular routine, and by meditation, which will help him relax and be more calm and patient. In addition, he and his partner might decide to spend more time on other aspects of lovemaking, which can last longer.

Couples need to understand and respect these differences. All too often, sexual differences between two people breed feelings of resentment or rejection. The partner who is more passionate feels rejected by the seemingly uninterested partner, while the one with the less insistent sex drive may resent the pressures of the more sexual one. To create harmony, each must bend toward the center to accommodate the other. From their increased understanding, they can work out a mutual compromise or adjustment, so that both can feel satisfied.

Five Ways to Build Intimacy in Your Relationship

In addition to the obvious solution of adjusting the frequency of lovemaking in a way that is mutually acceptable, another element in the accommodating process can be to find other ways of expressing intimacy. Many times, the perceived desire for sex stems from a different source: a desire for closeness, for love. This desire can be satisfied meaningfully through other expressions of intimacy.

The following suggestions do not come directly from any traditional Ayurvedic source, but they are very much in the spirit of Ayurveda, as their goal is the expansion of the heart. The one common denominator of these approaches is *time*: You must take some time to do them. Often there is a great deal of love in a relationship that doesn't come out simply because the partners don't take the time to express it. If you don't nourish the plant of your love, it will not blossom.

1. Cuddling. Spend some time, maybe half an hour to an hour, sitting or lying down together, just hugging and kissing and being close. See if you can do it without drifting off into talking and without letting it escalate into passion. Just share the closeness.

2. Feel your love. Sit or lie close to each other, with eyes closed, and silently feel the ways you love and appreciate each other. What are the qualities you admire in your partner, his or her special gifts, abilities, or ways that mean the most to you? Kindness, generosity, a sense of humor, wisdom, hard work, thriftiness, orderliness, a sense of adventure, responsibility, exuberance, steadiness—the possibilities are endless. If you are having trouble in your relationship and can't easily think of positive things about your partner, think back to what it was that drew you together in the first place.

3. Express your appreciation. Open your eyes and give verbal expression to what you felt in exercise 2—the love you feel for each other, the things you cherish and appreciate in each other. The easiest way is for one person to talk for a little while, then let the other talk. You saw how well this exercise worked with John and Anne in the previous chapter; it brought them to tears and a deep remembrance and renewal of the beauty of their original relationship.

4. Massage. Give each other a massage, in a loving but non-sexually stimulating way. Try to let the massage be an experience in itself, a giving and receiving of love, rather than a prelude to sex.

5. Communicate. Healthy communication promotes intimacy. Speak freely with each other about any blocks in your relationship that you would like to remove, such as any fear or insecurity that you may feel, or hopes for the relationship that have not yet been fulfilled. Or just share important recent feelings and thoughts of your own with your partner.

In general, keeping secrets from each other generates mistrust and creates distance. Sharing our inner secrets or experiences with a loved one can bring immense relief and promote the feeling of deep connectedness. It is amazing how love can begin to flow more freely after a good heart-to-heart talk.

These five exercises can substitute for sexual activity when that is desired, but they will also enhance your lovemaking when it occurs. That's because they increase intimacy, closeness, and love—the essential base for enjoying truly rewarding sex.

How to Overcome Society's Standards and Accept Your Own Sexuality

The lesson to be learned from the varying levels of sexuality among the constitutional types is that different degrees of interest in sex are not only legitimate and acceptable, they are *entirely normal.* Just as it wouldn't be healthy for everyone to have the same kind of daily diet or to do the same amount of vigorous exercise, it also isn't healthy to hold everyone to a single standard of sexual activity.

But because of our society's heavy emphasis on sex, many people feel there is something wrong with them if they don't have a hyperactive libido. Unfortunately, instead of helping these people toward self-acceptance, the medical profession often corroborates their feeling. "We need to get you more sexual," a therapist might say to such a person. "We need to put you in a class where you will masturbate, or watch sex movies, to give you a more 'normal' sex drive."

From an Ayurvedic point of view, this is usually not good advice. First of all, Ayurvedic texts unanimously state that masturbation tends to be physiologically unbalancing for two primary reasons, which have to do with ideal health and are not meant as moral judgments:

1. Masturbating aggravates Vata dosha, which could lead to insomnia and other Vata disorders such as anxiety, restlessness, and lack of ability to focus.
2. The expenditure of sexual energy, without the emotional bonding and energy exchange that take place in a loving relationship, also tends to create imbalance.

More important, the idea of trying to make all people conform to one standard of sexuality that does not take constitutional differences into account is extremely shortsighted and can do real harm. That's because many people, measuring themselves against the standard, feel that they are less than "okay."

If they don't have as strong a sexual drive as their spouse or partner, many men and women feel inadequate. Rebecca, for example, was seriously afraid there was something wrong with her because she didn't feel inclined toward lovemaking nearly as much as Steve was. After all, she was 32 years old, supposedly in the prime of her sexual life, yet most of the time she just didn't feel like having intercourse. She loved Steve, and they had what she considered "good sex" together, so she thought the fact that she didn't want to make love as much as he did was somehow her fault.

Unfortunately, Steve also thought it was her fault. He knew Rebecca enjoyed their lovemaking, and he didn't understand why she seemed to avoid it. She began to resent Steve for being "after her" all the time; Steve resented her for denying what he felt were normal and legitimate desires. Then after a while, her attitude made him fear that he *was* oversexed and demanding.

Tension built up between them. Rebecca felt, "I'm no good, I'm sexually inadequate," because of her low level of libido. But Steve also felt inadequate. The thought, "Maybe I can't perform well enough to please her" began to haunt him.

Fortunately, the solution was very simple—and you probably already know what it was. Steve was a Kapha-Pitta, and Rebecca a Vata-Pitta. The Pitta gave enough fire for their sexual encounters to be passionate and enjoyable, but the difference between the Kapha and the Vata caused the conflict. As soon as they understood this, they were able to relax, stop blaming each other, and develop a middle ground that was satisfying to both.

Examples like this show why it's so important to understand your constitution, to be alert to your own individual needs, and not to belittle yourself or think there's something wrong with you if you don't feel the same as the "standard." If, for example, you are feeling some draining effect from sex, then you need to respect and honor that sensitivity and understand that because of your constitutional type you have a limit as to what is good and healthful for you.

It is equally important to be sensitive to the sexual needs and desires of your partner and to be respectful of them if they are different from yours. The fact that there are differences doesn't mean that one of you is "right" and the other "wrong," that one is "healthy" and the other "unhealthy." That *may* be the case—but chances are that the differences are quite natural, and the key to harmony and mutual satisfaction is understanding.

Although this is standard knowledge in Ayurveda, it is not yet generally recognized or accepted in modern mental health circles or in medicine. In these circles, the prevailing attitude is that if you're having sex frequently, you're healthy; if less frequently, you're less healthy.

In Ayurveda, this is actually reversed. For reasons we shall explore in a moment, Ayurveda always recommends sex in moderation. Balance in this area is very important, and restraint is recommended, according to one's constitution. Obviously, what is "restraint" for a Kapha might feel like a wild honeymoon to a Vata; what is "restraint" for a Vata might feel like abstinence to a Kapha! But to whatever degree a person is comfortable, moderation is recommended.

"Less Is More"—When Less Lovemaking Is Better for You

To understand why this is so, we need to take another look at something we talked about in Chapter 5—the sequence of bodily processes that builds the seven basic tissues known as the dhatus. The reproductive tissue, shukra, is the seventh and last of these dhatus. Made of a refined material, it is vitally important for optimum functioning of our brain, nervous system, and immune system.

It is also a key factor for all kinds of creative expression and for the growth of consciousness toward enlightenment. In his book, *Prakruti: Your Ayurvedic Constitution,* Dr. Robert Svoboda writes,

> Shukra's functions are creation and creativity. Shukra can be used for procreation . . . or it can be used for the production of artistic or intellectual creations. . . . Weak Shukra means weak creativity.

When Shukra is released through sexual activity (particularly by the male in ejaculation), the amount of reproductive tissue is diminished. If this occurs too frequently for the individual, health problems could possibly result.

Shukra is also the basis of ojas, an even more refined product of the body that is sometimes referred to as the essence of life. Ayurvedic texts say that in the absence of ojas in the body, the person dies. An abundance of ojas gives vitality and power, love, joy, and an inner glow that radiates outward. Ojas gives a person a strong mind, flexible body, deep emotions, personal magnetism, and spiritual power.

From ancient times, the texts are specific about how to either increase or decrease this vital substance. The most important way to increase ojas is through deep meditation and the resultant experience of bliss that permeates the mind/body system. Conserving energy through decreased sexual activity is always recommended, as are eating certain foods, such as milk, ghee, rice, almonds, and honey.

Ojas is said to be diminished by excessive fasting or prolonged hunger; stress in the form of anxiety, fear, worry, or grief; overwork; too much sexual activity; hurry; excessive exposure to wind and sun; and staying up too late at night.

High levels of ojas build strong immunity. For that reason, Ayurveda closely links moderation in sex with better health. If sex is too frequent for a constitutional type, the immune system will become weaker. That may in turn give rise to increased susceptibility to infections such as colds, bronchitis, pneumonia, and other illnesses. Because sexual moderation increases the body's vitality, it is considered important for the successful treatment of many diseases.

Still another reason for moderation in sexual activity is that too frequent sex for any body type causes an aggravation of Vata. This can make a person susceptible to many diseases and problems that stem from unbalanced Vata.

Ayurveda suggests many ways to make it easier to naturally control sexual activity. Doing yoga exercises regularly, as well as meditation and breathing exercises can help in this regard. These practices promote a high degree of inner balance and satisfaction, which tends to decrease excessive cravings of all kinds.

In addition, certain foods and herbs are either recommended or proscribed. A person wishing to moderate sexual activity should abstain from red meat, garlic, and onions, as these foods stimulate the sexual appetite. Alcohol is also to be avoided. For a person who has a weak sexual drive that needs strengthening, these foods (but not the alcohol) might be helpful.

To help restore vitality after sexual intercourse, mix into a cup of warm milk a spoonful of ghee (clarified butter), a few ground-up almonds or cashews, and a teaspoon of raw sugar. A thread of saffron can also be added. The use of strengthening herbs such as winter cherry (ashvagandha) and Indian asparagus (shatavari) is also helpful.

Although the idea of sexual restraint as a key to spiritual development may be an unusual idea for you, the fact is that celibacy—total abstinence from sex—has been a central part of many of the world's monastic traditions for thousands of years. True, these are people who dedicate their entire lives to spiritual growth. But if you are a person seeking spiritual development, you may want the benefit of applying that powerful life energy to spiritual growth.

Techniques to help you sublimate and conserve that energy exist, available in numerous books and courses. Although not specifically from the Ayurvedic tradition, some Tantric teachings of India and Taoist teachings of China provide exercises, breathing practices, and other ways to help you enjoy the sexual experience without loss of energy. A book that might be useful if you are interested is *The Tao of Sexology* by Dr. Stephen T. Chang.

Gaining True Fulfillment

In our culture we generally tend to look outward for gratification: to our friends, families, lovers; to money and possessions that we can accumulate in order to have security; to new places we can live or visit; to entertainment we can lose ourselves in. This outward orientation—which is known as "object referral"—is all-pervasive in our society, and our attitude toward sex is colored by it.

For example, many people in our culture brag about their sexual conquests. This is about as self-centered and materialistic an attitude as a person could have: seeing other people as objects to be used for one's own pleasure.

The emphasis needs to be shifted from our endless fascination with objects to what Maharishi Ayur-Veda, in its strong emphasis on the importance of consciousness and inner development, calls "self-referral." Self-referral in its highest sense means looking inward to the ever-present bliss consciousness and unboundedness available on the quieter levels of awareness.

Practicing techniques of self-referral (especially meditation) regenerates our spirit and gives us more energy, happiness, and inner contentment. When we feel a greater sense of inner abundance, our behavior loses its needy, grasping quality and becomes spontaneously generous.

Outward achievements and enjoyments are never lasting, which is precisely why we become obsessed by them and addicted to them. Whether money, fame, food, alcohol, drugs, sex, the pursuit of it becomes addicting because the pleasure doesn't last, and one wants more. The preoccupation becomes a way to fill up an ever-emptying inner space. But fulfillment can never be gained from the outside, through the mechanism of trying to take in, in order to be filled.

Ayurveda in its deeper teachings holds that trying to gain lasting satisfaction through some outward behavior or activity, through a pill, or through connection with another person is a futile endeavor. Action, achievement, and relationship are certainly important parts of life, but deep, lasting fulfillment is gained within one's own self.

CHAPTER 19

AYURVEDIC SECRETS FOR HEALTHY PREGNANCY AND CHILDBIRTH

Modern medicine is just beginning to understand and to study the fact that there are countless influences on a child long before he or she is born. The genes inherited from both parents are important, but the influences on the child while in the womb are also very crucial to his or her future development. Here again, Ayurveda has much to teach us; thousands of years ago these influences were described in detail in the classic Ayurvedic texts.

Western obstetric care essentially begins with the verification of pregnancy and ends when the mother and her newborn infant are discharged from the hospital. By contrast, Ayurvedic care begins *before conception* and continues for the first several months of the child's life.

In this chapter we'll take a look at some of the traditional Ayurvedic recommendations both to ensure your baby's health and optimum development and to help *you* as well. These simple tips will keep you strong and balanced during pregnancy and will help you quickly regain the strength you'll need to care for your baby after delivery.

What to Do Before Conception

Ayurveda teaches that the influences on a child begin before conception, with the health of the father and mother. The classical texts state that it is vital for both parents to prepare themselves for the intended pregnancy. The quality of the sperm and egg, they say, will be maximized by healthy parents who are not stressed. The strength and purity of the parents will give the child a healthy constitution. It's like the old saying: "Well begun is half done."

Even the *intentions* of the parents are considered to be important. The ancient texts view having a child as a great event, not to be generated by a spontaneous act of passion, but by a carefully considered, conscious sequence of actions. First, the parents should envision the kind of child they want to have. As Robert Svoboda writes, freely paraphrasing the ancient Ayurvedic physician Charaka,

> A couple ought to want the strongest, most attractive, healthiest, highest-minded, highest-souled child who has ever popped out of the human mold, and should organize their lives to actualize this aim.

After praying for help,

> they should proceed elatedly and determinedly. After extensively purifying and rejuvenating their bodies, they should unite their seeds with joy and exultation on an auspicious night at an auspicious moment, to germinate a healthy embryo.

For about a year prior to conception, it is important for both parents to

- eat a pure, wholesome diet (emphasizing fresh foods and avoiding stale, canned, leftover, and packaged foods with additives, etc.)

- engage in a program for physical purification
- meditate regularly to reduce stress
- do daily oil massage
- use herbs and herbal supplements for additional nourishment and strengthening (such as *chyavanprash*, *Maharishi Amrit Kalash*, and herbs such as *ashvagandha* (winter cherry—especially for men) and *shatavari* (Indian asparagus—especially for women).

Restricted sexual activity, particularly during the last month or two before the desired conception, is also highly recommended. This is said to strengthen the seed, especially of the father, so as to impart more life energy and vitality (ojas) to the child.

The feelings of both parents at the time of conception are also considered very important in the formation of the child's character. Love, tenderness, and elevated, spiritual feelings are to be fostered as much as possible.

How to Help Your Child During Your Pregnancy

According to Ayurveda, the child in the womb is a living, conscious, sensitive being. This is particularly true after about three months, when the heart begins to beat and the child starts to kick and move. It is vitally important to expose the child, even in the womb, to wholesome foods and refined, positive attitudes and influences. The mother's diet, lifestyle, and emotions all play a big part in the development of her child's character, as well as his or her physical strength and health.

Since your child is basically eating what you eat and feeling what you feel, pregnant women who want the best for their children need to choose their food carefully, keep watch over their feelings, and live in a balanced, uplifting way.

Your diet should consist of the purest, freshest foods you can afford to buy. It should include lots of fresh (not canned or frozen) vegetables and fruits, whole grains, milk, almonds, fresh juices, ghee, and lots of water. Avoid junk food, alcohol, caffeine, and meat. Remember, if you eat junk food, that is what you are feeding your child. If you smoke, or drink alcohol, or use drugs, or breathe a lot of smog, so does your child. We have all seen the tragic stories of children born addicted to cocaine or other drugs because their mothers were addicted. Whatever is in your body, whether pure or impure, goes directly to your child.

Research also suggests that whatever rhythms the pregnant mother-to-be lives by, the child adopts as its own. If she meditates every afternoon at 3 o'clock, after birth her child, accustomed to that refreshing wave of deep rest, will tend to nap regularly at 3 o'clock. So a regular daily routine (see Chapter 6) is highly recommended.

Events in the environment also play a key role in the child's future development. There's a great deal of scientific evidence now that children are quite conscious during their stay in the womb and react to what goes on around them. Just as they absorb the foods and chemicals that the mother ingests, they also absorb emotions. That is why a harmonious environment, full of love, is so important. The child in the womb needs to be exposed to positive emotions and interactions. Violent films or movies that elicit feelings of fear are particularly not recommended, as are loud music or other noise. Arguments, fear, and all negativity are to be avoided.

Here the role of the husband is crucial. Ayurveda emphasizes that it is the husband's job to provide as much emotional nourishment and love to his pregnant wife as possible. Although many women don't like to admit it, most strongly desire to feel added protection, support, and affection from their mates during these months. Husbands need to stay home as much as possible in the evenings and take on more responsibility for the household chores and care of the other children, if there are any.

Here is a summary of the Ayurvedic guidelines for a most successful pregnancy:

- Walk for about half an hour every day. If you are accustomed to more vigorous exercise, swimming is acceptable, but it's best not to run, lift, or strain.
- If you have been doing the Sun Salutation and Yoga Postures, it's best to stop doing them during pregnancy.
- *Go to bed early and get lots of rest*—very crucial!
- Pay attention to your diet. Have nourishing meals at regular intervals. Food should be warm and well-cooked for easy diges-

tion. With moderation, lean toward the Vata-pacifying diet, no matter what your body type. If Vata is aggravated in the mother during pregnancy, the child will be prone to fear, anxiety, and Vata disorders. Avoid much in the way of raw salads or beans (both Vata-aggravating), and also be moderate with hot, spicy foods.

Emphasize fresh fruit and vegetables, milk, honey, almonds (blanched is better), whole grains. As a group, food with the *sweet* taste is recommended; it has a strengthening, building-up quality. This includes bread, cereal and other grain products, milk, rice, and sweet fruits. It does *not* include refined sugar, which should be minimized. Butter and ghee are excellent now (but not to extremes).

- As always, avoid canned and frozen food, leftovers, and food with chemical additives such as preservatives and artificial color and flavor.

- Food cravings may be more than just amusing—they may signal your own body's attempts at balance or may even indicate something your baby needs for proper development. Use common sense to evaluate them, but in general tend to trust your cravings and to satisfy them.

- Daily meditation is very helpful during pregnancy. Many women have reported that it is relaxing and soothing and relieves stress.

- Daily oil massage is also very soothing and nourishing. Be very gentle in massaging the abdominal area.

- Mother should experience as little stress as possible. No violent movies, loud music, conflicts and arguments, or harsh environments. The child feels it all.

- Surround yourself with positive influences and beauty. Read uplifting books, watch videos that have a positive quality. Be with people you love and who love you. Play beautiful, soothing music. If you can, have some flowers in the house and sweet fragrances in the form of incense or fragrant oils.

- Be happy. The more happiness the mother experiences, the more her baby will be blissful and happy. Your biochemistry is transferred to your child. As much as practically possible, avoid anything that makes you unhappy.

- In the eighth and ninth month, rest as much as you can.

Secrets for Healthy Childbirth

If a woman has followed these guidelines, especially maintaining a restful, low-stress routine, paying proper attention to diet, and getting some regular exercise during pregnancy, her chances of a comfortable birth are increased. Here are some tips to make the birth process easier and more comfortable for both mother and baby:

- The surroundings are important. If you can, arrange to have the birth in a comfortable room, with subdued lighting and soft, pleasant music, rather than on an operating table under bright glaring lights.
- Have some company, preferably a woman you know and trust. Many women like to have their husbnds with them at this time. Research is corroborating that women who have a companion—have fewer complications, shorter labor, and seem to feel better and happier afterwards.
- Deep breathing is helpful to keep Vata in balance.
- Remember that any medications the mother takes are also taken by the baby.

After the Baby is Born—Ayurvedic Tips for Mom

Well, Mom, congratulations—you made it through pregnancy (morningsickness, backaches, the whole deal), through labor, and through delivery. And there's your beautiful new baby! But guess what—this is where the hard part starts. Get ready for middle-of-the-night feedings and a schedule worse than a medical student's.

Luckily, Ayurveda has a host of suggestions to help you in these next weeks and months. If you follow them, you will feel much better, much stronger and will have more love to offer your child. If you've had children before and follow these guidelines with a new baby, you will immediately see and feel the difference.

First of all, you need to get extra rest. You've got to restructure your life and slow down so that you're not constantly on the run. How can you do this when you now have even *more* to deal with? Only one way: You've got to get some help. Whether it comes from your husband or from older children taking on some added responsibility, or from other family members, friends, or some hired short-term help, you need to cut back on your workload for at least the first month or two. Cooking, cleaning, shopping, and other chores need to be handled by someone else as much as possible.

Going back to work is your decision; you may feel you have to, in order not to lose a job you need to keep. But for your own sake and your baby's, Ayurveda would definitely recommend taking a leave of absence of at least several months if at all possible.

One suggestion from Maharishi Ayur-Veda for your daily routine is that at least once a day, when your baby naps, rather than trying to use that time to do chores you should also lie down and take a nap. This will help you make up for some of the sleep you lose at night and for some of the fatigue caused by your very irregular schedule.

Next to getting extra rest, your main need will be to balance Vata. Vata governs motion, and the intense activity in the body during delivery greatly accentuates this dosha. Then, following the birth, you will encounter more Vata-disrupting factors. Schedule irregularity, lost sleep, exhaustion, are all Vata-aggravating. The common experience of post-partum depression is largely caused by aggravated Vata.

Therefore what you need is a comprehensive Vata-pacifying program. Here are the main components:

- Extra rest is vital, as I've suggested.
- A daily oil massage, even for five minutes, will be very helpful. (See instructions in Chapter 4.)
- Follow your oil massage with a warm bath. Try to soak for at least five to ten minutes, just letting yourself relax.
- Daily meditation will be rejuvenating and relaxing.
- Now is the time to start doing the Yoga Postures and Sun Salutation again—but go very easy at the start and break back in slowly.
- For some light aerobic exercise, a daily walk of about 15 to 30 minutes will be ideal.
- Follow the Vata-pacifying diet. Guidelines are in Chapter 3, but the basics include an emphasis on warm, cooked foods such

as soups and stews, rice and wheat products, well-cooked fresh vegetables, sweet, juicy fruit (not dried), and plenty of dairy products, especially milk and ghee. You can have oily, but not fried foods. Almonds, which are said to increase breast milk, are a good snack. Warm rice pudding with milk and un-refined sugar is an excellent, strengthening treat. Favor the sweet, sour, and salty tastes and avoid pungent, bitter, and as-tringent.

- Use the herb shatavari (Indian asparagus). It is a rejuvenative herb for the female reproductive system and is said to increase breast milk. You can take capsules, boil some powder in water and drink as a tea, or use as much as 3 grams (1 tsp) in warm milk with some natural unrefined sugar.

Ayurvedic Tips for Your Baby's First Weeks

Your baby girl has just come from nine months in a quiet, protected environment. She doesn't want to go to parties or ride on the sub-way; she needs to be safeguarded for some time from harsh stimuli in the environment such as loud noises or bright lights. Ayurveda actually recommends keeping your newborn indoors for about six weeks, except for occasional short walks in mild weather. Watch out for cold drafts, both indoors and out.

Breast feeding is strongly recommended for at least the first six months. Nancy Lonsdorf, M.D., one of the authors of *A Woman's Best Medicine,* suggests breast feeding "on demand" for two weeks, then gradually modifying it to at least two-hour intervals. Weaning can begin after six to eight months when your child's teeth begin to appear and should be completed by the age of 18 months.

If positive impressions were important during the prenatal pe-riod, they are certainly important now. The child has what the edu-cator Maria Montessori called "an absorbent mind," which soaks up everything in the environment and "metabolizes" it, making it part of his or her nature.

Daily sesame oil massage (see box) will be relaxing and help your baby sleep and digest better. It also aids circulation and breathing.

HOW TO GIVE YOUR INFANT A SOOTHING, ENLIVENING MASSAGE

One of the most wonderful things you can do for your baby is a daily oil massage, similar to the one you give to yourself. The massage will not only be very soothing and relaxing, it also helps improve immunity and circulation.

First carefully read the directions in Chapter 4; modify the instructions slightly as needed to care for your very delicate child.

- Use warm sesame oil—careful, not too hot!
- Use only a small amount of oil for the entire massage.
- Hold the baby on your lap or place him or her on a pillow covered in plastic.
- Begin with the head; be very gentle with the fontanelles (soft spots) on top of the head. Avoid eyes and skip inside ears.
- Motions are similar to those for an adult—circular motions on joints, straight back and forth motions on long bones.
- Spend a couple of minutes making long, gentle strokes up and down the back, and a minute or so on the soles of the feet.
- Entire massage should take about five to ten minutes.
- After the massage, wash the baby in mild soap and warm water. *Be extra careful*—the oil will make your baby very slippery.

Note: A videotape entitled *Blissful Baby: The Maharishi Ayur-Vedic Mother/Baby Program* shows in detail how to perform the baby massage and includes a wealth of other information for both mother and baby, including suggestions for feeding, exercising the infant, and weaning. It is available at Maharishi Ayur-Veda Medical Centers (see Appendix B).

There is no time more tender and delicate than the first few months of life. The guidelines in this chapter can help any mother give the most to her baby during this period, while also taking the best care of herself. By getting extra rest and bringing her body quickly back into balance after the child is born, she will be able to give more relaxed, loving attention to her child and have some left over for the rest of her family.

CHAPTER 20

AYURVEDA AND THE FUTURE OF MEDICINE

The worldwide revival of the ancient Ayurvedic system of natural healing is helping to transform the shape of modern medicine. Among the many ways in which Ayurveda is bringing vital new life to medical theory and practice, there are three I'd like to mention.

1. *A new emphasis on prevention.* Medicine today has been focused almost exclusively on what we might call "disease care" rather than on health care. Our ability to treat many illnesses is highly developed, but almost no attention is paid to *preventing* illness. Ayurveda, with its strong emphasis on utilizing diet, exercise, and other natural strategies to maintain and improve health, is helping to change that.

2. *Personal responsibility for health.* Many people today are realizing that responsible health care is up to us. By the choices we make every day, we choose either health or illness. If we get enough rest, nourish ourselves with fresh, pure food and positive influences, if we get exercise suited to our constitution, we are creating health. If not, we are looking for trouble, and it will eventually find us.

This is borne out by the fact that even as science gets control of infectious diseases such as tuberculosis, smallpox, and so forth, other deadly illnesses such as cancer and heart disease are increasing, especially *in the developed nations of the world*. This indicates that these are *lifestyle* diseases, caused by the way we as individuals and as a society conduct our lives. Such factors as stress, smoking, air and water pollution, lack of exercise and poor diet, are making us sick.

Ayurveda offers hundreds of guidelines for living a long, healthy life in tune with nature. By putting some of these to use, we can take control of our own health.

3. *A unique program for global well-being.* Crime, violence, and war are not usually considered a problem of medicine and health, but in reality they are symptoms of a widespread epidemic of stress. Throughout the world, stress levels are climbing to new heights every day, due to economic pressures, the increasingly fast pace of life, the transformation of societies into the post-industrial age, the breakdown of families and moral values, and so on.

When stress builds up in us as individuals, it eventually explodes in anger. Just like that, crime, violence, and wars are due primarily to accumulated stress throughout society. Stress reduction through meditation and other modalities of Ayurveda offers a solution that deserves widespread and careful consideration for creating a better world.

Let's look a little more deeply at each of these three important ideas.

Prevention: The Medicine of the Future

If you examine our medical system today, you'll see big hospitals and HMOs, multimillion-dollar high-tech equipment, and thousands of expensive drugs. This system gobbles up hundreds of billions of dollars every year. It is called a "health care" system, but there is little evidence that as a society we are actually getting any healthier.

Actually, what we have is a "disease care" system; when we get sick, we enter that system for help. But what about a more important concern: What can we do to *stay* healthy?

If you have ever had any part in this system, either as a patient or as a medical professional, you will immediately realize that very little, *if any*, time and money are devoted to genuine prevention.

(What is called "prevention" usually involves testing—sometimes at considerable expense—to see if you have anything wrong with you.)

When were you given a set of practical, personalized guidelines for healthy living according to your individual constitution and circumstances? Where are the careful discussions between wise physicians and their patients, to ensure that each person is living in such as way as to remain in vibrant health?

That is what is needed today. Simply by intelligent, informed choices involving the basics of life—what to eat and how to eat, what kind of exercise is suited to you, how to structure your daily routine to help you attune to the powerful rhythms of nature, as well as other natural strategies—you can learn how to prevent imbalances from arising, and maintain good health year after year.

Prevention will surely be the emphasis of the medicine of the future. It's the only way that makes sense. Why should we allow ourselves to get sick, if it is possible to stay healthy? Why should we endure not only the discomforts or agonies of illness, but also the considerable inconvenience and high costs? The answer to the rising cost of health care is not placing limits on who gets what kind of care from whom—the current "managed care" debate in the United States—but true *prevention*. This will eliminate billions of dollars from the health care budget and will allow full care for everyone who does become sick and needs attention.

Prominent researchers have estimated that a 50 percent reduction in health care costs is very feasible through effective prevention programs. For example, research has been published on studies in the United States and Canada that show that people who practice Transcendental Meditation and other strategies of Maharishi Ayur-Veda have health care costs at least 50 percent lower than other people of the same age and background. Just getting people to quit smoking, do some moderate exercise a few times a week, eat less fat, and meditate for stress reduction would save the nation tens or even hundreds of billions of dollars every year, not to mention the enormous benefits to people's lives.

So you deserve congratulations! As a reader of this book, you are pioneering the new age of preventive medicine that is going to bring better health to everyone.

Take Charge of Your Own Well-Being

Now that infectious diseases such as tuberculosis and polio are largely under control around the world, we can all relax and enjoy perfect health and long life, right? Wrong! Other killer illnesses, such as heart disease and various forms of cancer, have increased tremendously in the United States and in other industrial and technologically advanced nations.

These diseases seem to be closely related to our way of life. High levels of stress, a diet far too heavy in animal fats, smoking, alcohol abuse, a sedentary lifestyle with little exercise—these factors are without a doubt the basic causes of most heart disease and are increasingly implicated in several of the most common types of cancer.

But here's the good news. Because these factors are largely within our control, these dread diseases are to a great extent preventable. A few simple lifestyle changes can make all the difference in the world.

From the Ayurvedic perspective, the key to maintaining excellent long-term health is to know how to keep your body and mind in balance. You need to know

- Your body type or constitution.
- The basics of diet and lifestyle that promote health for your constitution—good foods to eat, ideal daily routine, healthful environmental conditions, daily meditation, best type of exercise, etc.
- The risk factors for your constitution—wrong foods to eat, environmental conditions to avoid, exercise that would be either insufficient or excessive, etc.

These three factors can easily be learned from this book.

I would also suggest a fourth strategy, which I cannot teach you here—self pulse-diagnosis, so that you can monitor your day-to-day health, discover imbalances, and then take measures to correct them by regulating your diet and daily activities. This is an effortless and effective method of prevention. We have touched upon it briefly (page 30) but please see Appendix B for Ayurvedic medical centers where the art of pulse diagnosis can be learned in depth.

You can easily maintain excellent mental and physical health throughout your lifetime by learning and applying the principles of Ayurveda outlined in this book. It is my hope that you will put this great knowledge to use, for your own benefit and for the collective health of humanity.

The World is My Family: A Unique Approach to Creating a Healthy, Peaceful World

Ultimately, health is more than an individual issue. If you think about it, you can see that there is such a thing as a healthy or unhealthy relationship, family, or community. ·Nations, too, can be healthy or unhealthy, moral or immoral; they can have severe collective mental health problems, as witness the mass delusion and violence of Nazi Germany.

We can also speak of the mental health of the world. Even though massive anxiety, mutual fear and suspicion, ruthless competition, and war are widespread and common in the family of nations, they are actually all signs of mental disorder. On the other hand, peace, harmony, cooperation, and contentment would indicate balanced world consciousness, just as they are signs of individual health.

Although this seems obvious, it has seemed impractical to do much about it. Yet there are now studies indicating that there is a way to create a positive influence on the health of the environment.

In recent years, the *Journal of Conflict Resolution*, the *Journal of Mind and Behavior*, and other top-level scientific publications have reported on experiments in which a group of several thousand people was able to produce an influence of coherence and positivity on their surroundings. They did this by meditating together and in that way producing more coherent brain waves due to their calm, relaxed state of mind.

The studies showed that these groups of meditators, who were practicing the meditation techniques of Maharishi Ayur-Veda (Transcendental Meditation and the more advanced TM-Sidhi program), produced measurable and significant decreases in the incidence of crime, suicides, social turbulence, and international conflict. One study reported reduced conflict in the Middle East during the

Lebanon war in 1983, including a 75 percent reduction in war deaths when a large group convened for group practice of TM. In a 1993 experiment in Washington, D.C., a similar group reduced violent crime by nearly 20 percent in two months.

Another exciting area of social research is criminal rehabilitation. Numerous studies have now been published showing that introduction of TM into prison settings (including Folsom prison in California, the state prison system of Vermont, and the entire criminal justice system of the country of Senegal) results in very significant benefits, including decreased violence in the prison environment and enhanced moral development among the prisoners. Perhaps most importantly, the recidivism rate—the rate of return to prison of those who have been released—is greatly reduced, suggesting that effective rehabilitation has actually taken place.

Today, growing concern about the environment, global economic problems, deadly conflicts such as the Gulf War and the war in Bosnia continue to cause unhappiness and make us despair of ever creating a better world. These studies of the positive influence of group consciousness suggest a new approach to resolving both local and global problems by increasing coherence in the world's atmosphere. They offer hope of a world that is genuinely healthy, happy, cooperative, and harmonious.

That would be the fulfillment of an ancient saying from the Vedic tradition that gave rise to Ayurveda: *The world is my family.* It would be wonderful if in our lifetime we could see a genuine world peace, made possible at last through elimination of stress and the creation of global coherence.

For Further Reading About Ayurveda

Books

Ayurveda: The Science of Self-Healing, Dr. Vasant Lad (Santa Fe: Lotus Press, 1984).

The Yoga of Herbs: An Ayurvedic Guide to Herbal Medicine, Dr. Vasant Lad and Dr. David Frawley (Santa Fe: Lotus Press, 1986).

Perfect Health, Deepak Chopra, M.D. (New York: Harmony, 1990).

A Woman's Best Medicine: Health, Happiness, and Long Life Through Maharishi Ayur-Veda, Nancy Lonsdorf, M.D., Veronica Butler, M.D., and Melanie Brown, Ph.D.

Ayurveda: Life, Health and Longevity, Dr. Robert Svoboda (London: Arkana, 1992).

Prakruti: Your Ayurvedic Constitution, Dr. Robert Svoboda (Albuquerque: Geocom, 1989).

Ayurvedic Healing: A Comprehensive Guide, Dr. David Frawley (Salt Lake City: Passage Press, 1989).

The Book of Ayurveda, Judith M. Morrison (New York: Fireside, 1995).

Ayurvedic Cooking for Self-Healing, Dr. Vasant Lad and Usha Lad (Albuquerque: The Ayurvedic Press, 1994).

The Ayurvedic Cookbook, Amadea Morningstar (Santa Fe: Lotus Press, 1990).

Body, Mind and Sport, Dr. John Douillard (New York: Harmony, 1992).

Correspondence Courses

A course in the basics of Ayurveda by Dr. Robert Svoboda is available through The Ayurvedic Institute in Albuquerque (see address and phone in Appendix B).

A course by Dr. David Frawley is available through the American Institute of Vedic Studies, P.O. Box 8357, Santa Fe, NM 87504, telephone (505) 983-9385.

AYURVEDA TREATMENT AND TEACHING CENTERS AND PHYSICIANS

The Ayurvedic Institute
P.O. Box 23445
Albuquerque, NM 87192-1445
(505) 291-9698

Training programs, seminars, private consultations (by appointment only), panchakarma treatments, and an herb department. The director of the Institute is Dr. Vasant Lad.

Maharishi Ayur-Veda Colleges, Schools and Health Centers Offer training programs, private consultations, panchakarma treatments, herbs (by prescription), and other programs.

281

Following are the addresses of four main treatment centers for Maharishi Ayur-Veda. In addition several hundred physicians and other health care practitioners have been trained in Maharishi Ayur-Veda. You can contact these health professionals through these four centers.

The Raj
1734 Jasmine Ave.
Fairfield, IA 52556
800-248-9050

Maharishi Ayur-Veda Medical
  Center
17308 Sunset Blvd.
Pacific Palisades, CA 90272
310-454-5531

Nancy Lonsdorf, M.D.
Maharishi Ayur-Veda Medical
  Center
4910 Massachusetts Ave., N.W.
Suite 315
Washington, D.C. 20016
202-244-2700

Maharishi Ayur-Veda Medical
  Center
679 George Hill Road
Lancaster, MA 01523
508-365-4549

The following practitioners have received traditional training in Ayurvedic natural medicine.

Dr. Lobsang Rapgay
2206 Benecia Avenue
West Los Angeles, CA 90064
310-282-9918

Dr. Satnam S. Sandhu
Apt #2, 68 Montgomery St.
Bloomfield, NJ 07003
201-743-1758

Acharya A. L. Metha
7806 Galveston Road
Houston, Texas
713-947-7348 or
    713-947-4647

Ayurvedic & Naturopathic
  Medical Clinic
Dr. Virender Sodhi
10025 N.E. 4th St.
Bellevue, WA 98004
206-453-8022

Dr. Vivek Shanbag
144 NE 54th St.
Seattle, WA 98105
206-523-9585

Dr. Sukumaran
5526 SE Marine Dr.
Burnaby B.C. Canada V5J3G8
    (near Vancouver)
604-431-0950

Academy of Ayurveda: Natural
    Health Care Center
Dr. Surendra N. Tripathi,
    Director
2558 Danforth Ave., Suite 202
Toronto, Ontario
Canada M4C 1L3
416-691-6841

WHERE TO OBTAIN AYURVEDIC HERBS, TEAS, ETC.

Most of the common herbs and some of the special Indian herbs used in Ayurveda and mentioned in this book can be easily obtained in bulk or capsules at natural food stores in most cities throughout the country.

Other Sources

The Ayurvedic Institute
P.O. Box 23445
Albuquerque, NM 87192-1445
(505) 291-9698

A large selection of herbs, herbal compounds, and tinctures under the supervision of Dr. Vasant Lad.

283

Bazaar of India Imports, Inc.
1810 University Avenue
Berkeley, CA 94703
1-800-261-7662; (510) 548-4110

A large selection of herbs in bulk at excellent prices. Free catalogue
on request.

Maharishi Ayurveda Products International
P.O. Box 49667
Colorado Springs, CO 80949
1-800-843-8332 or 1-800-255-8332

Use this source for Maharishi Ayur-Veda products mentioned in this
book, such as Maharishi Amrit Kalash and Vata, Pitta, and Kapha
teas and churnas. Numerous other products are available. Free catalogue on request.

Kanak
P.O. Box 13653
Albuquerque, NM 87192-3653

Ayurvedic preparations unavailable elsewhere.

SELECTED BIBLIOGRAPHY, SCIENTIFIC RESEARCH ON TRANSCENDENTAL MEDITATION AND MAHARISHI AYUR-VEDA

Bleick, C. R., and A. I. Abrams. 1987. The Transcendental Meditation program and criminal recidivism in California. *The Journal of Criminal Justice* 15: 211–30.

Brooks, J. S., and T. Scarano. 1985. Transcendental Meditation in the treatment of post-Vietnam adjustment. *Journal of Counseling and Development* 65: 212–15.

Chandler, H. M., D. W. Orme-Johnson, M. C. Dillbeck, and J. L. Glaser. June 1985. Improvements in memory, intelligence, psychomotor speed, and alertness in normal subjects from an Ayur-Vedic medicinal herbal-based rejuvenation therapy. Paper presented at the Twenty-eighth Annual Meeting of the Society of Economic Botany, University of Illinois, Chicago.

Cooper, M. J., and M. M. Aygen. 1987. Effect of Transcendental Meditation on serum cholesterol and blood pressure. *Harefuah* (journal of the Israel Medical Association) 95: 1–2.

Dillbeck, M. C., and D. W. Orme-Johnson. 1987. Physiological differences between Transcendental Meditation and rest. *American Psychologist* 42: 879–81.

Dillbeck, M. C., K. L. Cavanaugh, T. Glenn, D. W. Orme-Johnson, and V. Mittlefehldt. 1987. Consciousness as a field: The Transcendental Meditation and TM-Sidhi program and changes in social indicators. *The Journal of Mind and Behaviour* 8: 67–104.

Dwivedi, C., B. Satter, and H. M. Sharma. 1991. Anticarcinogenic activity of an Ayur-Vedic food supplement. Maharishi Amrit Kalash (MAK). *Pharmacology, Biochemistry and Behavior* 39: 649–52.

Eppley, K., A. Abrams, and J. Shear. 1989. Differential effects of relaxation techniques on trait anxiety: A meta-analysis. *Journal of Clinical Psychology* 45: 957–74.

Fields, J. Z., et al. 1990. Oxygen free radical scavenging effects of an anticarcinogenic natural product, Maharishi Amrit Kalash (MAK). *American Society for Pharmacology and Experimental Therapeutics* 32: 55.

Gelderloos, P., K. Walton, and D. W. Orme-Johnson. 1990. Effectiveness of the Transcendental Meditation program in preventing and treating substance abuse: A review. *International Journal of the Addictions* 26: 293–325.

Kasture, H. S., S. Rothenberg, R. Averbach, K. Cavanaugh, D. K. Robinson, and R. K. Wallace. September 1985. Improvements in mental and physical health with the Maharishi Ayur-Veda Panchakarma program. Paper presented at the Eighth World Congress of the International College of Psychosomatic Medicine, Chicago.

Orme-Johnson, D. W. 1988. Medical care utilization and the Transcendental Meditation program. *Psychosomatic Medicine* 49: 493–500.

Schneider, R. H., R. K. Wallace, H. S. Kasture, R. Averbach, S. Rothenberg, and D. R. Robinson. 1990. Physiological and psychological correlates of Maharishi Ayur-Veda psychosomatic types. *Journal of Social Behavior and Personality* 5: 1–27.

Sharma, H. M., C. Dwivedi, B. C. Satter, H. A. Gudehitihlu, W. Malarkey, and G. A. Tejwani. 1990. Antineoplastic properties of Maharishi-4, against

DMBA-induced mammary tumors in rats. *Journal of Pharmacy, Biochemistry and Behavior* 35: 767–73.

Stryker, T., and R. K. Wallace. September 1985. Reduction in biological age through an Ayur-Vedic treatment program. Paper presented to the International Congress of Psychosomatic Medicine, Chicago.

Wallace, R. K., M. C. Dillbeck, E. Jacobe, and B. Harrington. 1982. The effects of the Transcendental Meditation and TM-Sidhi program on the aging process. *International Journal of Neuroscience* 16: 53–58.

Wallace, R. K., J. Silver, P. Mills, M. C. Dillbeck, and D. E. Wagner. 1983. Systolic blood pressure and long-term practice of the Transcendental Meditation and TM-Sidhi program: Effects of TM on systolic blood pressure. *Psychosomatic Medicine* 45: 41–46.

For information on current research on Maharishi Ayur-Veda, please contact:

The Institute of Science, Technology and Public Policy
1000 N. 4th St.
Fairfield, Iowa 52557-1137
(515) 472-1200
Fax: (515) 472-1165

INDEX